CLINICAL ANATOMY
OF THE DOG & CAT

A Color Atlas of

CLINICAL ANATOMY OF THE DOG & CAT

J S Boyd
BVMS PhD MRCVS
Professor of Veterinary Anatomy
The University of Glasgow Veterinary School
Bearsden, Glasgow

C Paterson
MSc
Research Technician
Department of Veterinary Anatomy
The University of Glasgow Veterinary School
Bearsden, Glasgow

A H Msay
ARPS AMPA
Head Photographer
Department of Photography
The University of Glasgow Veterinary School
Bearsden, Glasgow

Ｍ Mosby-Wolfe

A CIP catalogue record is available from the British Library

Print number   10 9 8 7 6 5 4 3
© Copyright J.S. Boyd and C. Paterson, 1991
Published by Wolfe Publishing Ltd, 1991
Reprinted in 1995 by Mosby–Wolfe, an imprint of Times Mirror International Publishers Limited
Printed by BPCC Hazell Ltd, Aylesbury, Bucks., England

For full details of all Mosby–Year Book Europe Limited titles please write to Mosby–Year Book Europe Limited, Lynton House, 7–12 Tavistock Square, London WC1H 9LB, England.
A CIP catalogue record for this book is available from the British Library.

Contents

Preface

Instruction in veterinary anatomy is usually approached in one of two ways: in the initial stages of undergraduate teaching, the emphasis is mainly on structure and function, with a demand for greater detail of the individual organs, usually presented on a systems basis. At this stage, students use the standard texts that rely on illustrating the anatomical features by means of line diagrams. Later in their studies, the students become more aware of the importance of regional and topographical anatomy, where line diagrams may not fully illustrate the structures seen during dissection or clinical examination. For this reason, the greater topographical detail of a pictorial atlas is often preferred.

Veterinary anatomical atlases, past and present, have followed the conventions of human anatomical teaching, using either detailed artists' impressions or photographs of embalmed, dissected cadavers. The lack of realism, with the loss of normal colour and form, often detracts from these publications, as the specimens demonstrated so often bear little resemblance to the natural organs and tissues. Veterinary anatomy differs widely from its human counterpart in its ability to utilise fresh material. The veterinary clinician, surgeon or pathologist would much prefer to consult an anatomy atlas that presents with greater realism those structures encountered when examining or operating on a living animal, or when performing an autopsy. Greater demands are also being made of anatomical teaching to accommodate the newer imaging modalities, such as radiography and ultrasonography, where topographical and cross-sectional anatomy is becoming increasingly relevant.

This atlas provides photographic illustrations of the gross anatomy of the dog and cat, using, wherever possible, fresh, unprocessed material. Bony specimens have been presented in a more classical anatomical fashion, but they are displayed both singly and in articulated form, with areas of muscle attachment clearly outlined. The book begins with the head and works logically, on a regional basis, in a caudal direction. The osteology of each region is illustrated and the topography of the organs and structures is revealed, first in terms of living surface anatomy and then through a series of prepared dissections of fresh cadavers. The salient structures that appear in the photographs are numbered to correspond to the legends in order to assist identification, and also to facilitate self testing by the reader. Wherever pertinent, clinical and surgical features of note are also described alongside the photographs to enlarge upon the illustrated structures and regions. The degree of detail in the presentation of the vascular and neural supplies is deliberately restricted: only major vessels and nerve trunks are named when they are of particular interest in surgical fields or are of clinical importance. The radiographic features of each region are displayed and cross-sectional anatomical specimens are used, where appropriate, to demonstrate particular topographical planes. In certain regions, ultrasonographs of soft tissue structures are used for comparison with the cross-sectional anatomy.

Most of the photographs and the text refer to the anatomy of the dog, while cat anatomy is given a more comparative role, with morphological differences between the species being illustrated. The dissections have been prepared from fresh material, but all the cadavers used for the photographs were animals that had to undergo euthanasia for other reasons. No animal was sacrificed to provide illustrative material for this publication.

With the dissections, the policy has been to reveal structures in as natural a manner as possible: thus realism has been a greater consideration than stylised anatomical preparation. This type of approach has produced a veterinary anatomical atlas that shows that veterinary anatomy need no longer be limited to the examination of artificially prepared, embalmed specimens, but that it can serve the needs of those requiring realistic anatomical information when studying or practising veterinary medicine.

6

Acknowledgements

The authors would most sincerely like to thank Allan May, whose great skill as a photographer made the production of this book possible. His endless patience and sense of humour brought pleasure to otherwise difficult and sometimes disappointing tasks.

The radiographs of the thorax, abdomen and spinal column were provided by radiographer Janice Lloyd, DCR, to whom we are indebted. The bone preparations were produced by Susan Cain, whom we thank for her skill and perseverance.

We also wish to extend our gratitude to our respective wives, Isobel and Jean, for their forbearance and encouragement throughout the long hours of preparation of this book.

J S Boyd
C Paterson

Dedication

To the memory of the late Helen J Smith,
MRCVS, former Head of the Department of
Veterinary Anatomy at Glasgow University
Veterinary School, who gave us our initial
and lasting enthusiasm for the study of
veterinary anatomy.

1 Introduction

Without wishing to appear too pedantic, the consistent use of basic anatomical terminology is of paramount importance to permit proper communication not only among veterinary anatomists themselves, but also between anatomists and clinicians. To this end, a common nomenclature has been devised, *Nomina Anatomica Veterinaria* (NAV), that has greatly assisted in clarifying the channels of communication.

At first sight, the system may seem laboured, since the original NAV is in Latin, but it is quite permissible to use the same terms and names translated into English, as happens in many instances throughout the atlas. However, where muscles of the body appear in key lists, the Latin form has been retained to avoid a conflict in terminology. On a few occasions, an alternative term may appear after the standard NAV version, where an older name for a structure is still so widely used that it is regarded as common parlance.

When discussing topographical anatomy, the need for uniform description of both direction and position also becomes obvious. The photographs of the live dog in this chapter are annotated to demonstrate the standard directional and positional terms (**1–3**). Also included are a small number of regional names for specific areas of the body and limbs. Adjectives that have common usage in human anatomy, such as 'anterior', 'posterior', 'superior' and 'inferior', should not be employed in veterinary anatomy, except in a limited number of instances, to describe certain structures in the head region (e.g., within the eye or the brain).

In the live animal, standing erect on all four limbs, structures located towards the back (*dorsum*) of the animal are said to be 'dorsal' in position; this applies to the trunk, head and even the tail. The opposite of this position is termed 'ventral', describing structures that lie closest to the belly (*venter*) of the animal. Any structures that are located towards the head (*cranium*) are referred to as 'cranial', while those located towards the tail (*cauda*) are said to be

'caudal'. This system of identification requires finer definition in the head region itself, where the term 'rostral' is used for structures located closer to the muzzle (*rostrum*), rather than the broader term 'cranial'. However, the contrary direction in the head region is still termed 'caudal'.

The median (*medianus*) plane passes through the animal from head to tail, along the line of the vertebral column (*axis*), and divides the whole body into two symmetrical halves. Planes passing to either side of the median plane but parallel to it are referred to as 'sagittal'. However, sometimes, if the plane is close to the median, it is called 'paramedian'. The structures that lie closer to the median plane are said to be 'medial', while those that lie towards the outer side or flank (*latus*) of the animal are classified as 'lateral'. Sections of the head and trunk, that are parallel to the back (*dorsum*) of the animal are said to be in the dorsal plane, whereas sections made at right angles to the axis of the body are referred to as being 'transverse'.

The limbs require further definition and interpretation because their position may alter relative to the trunk. The proximal region of a limb is that closer to the trunk, while the area further from the trunk is distal. In the proximal region of the thoracic and pelvic limbs (i.e., down to the proximal limit of the carpus and tarsus) the area closer to the 'front' of the limb is cranial in contrast to the area closer to the 'rear', which is caudal. Distal to the carpus in the thoracic limb, the continuation of the cranial surface is termed 'dorsal' and that of the caudal surface is 'palmar'. With the pelvic limb, the equivalent terms for areas distal to the tarsus are 'dorsal' and 'plantar'. There is also a notional central axis running the length of each limb, and any section perpendicular to it is termed 'transverse'. If a structure in the limb lies closer to the central axis, it is 'axial' in position, in contrast to structures lying away from the central axis, which are 'abaxial'.

1

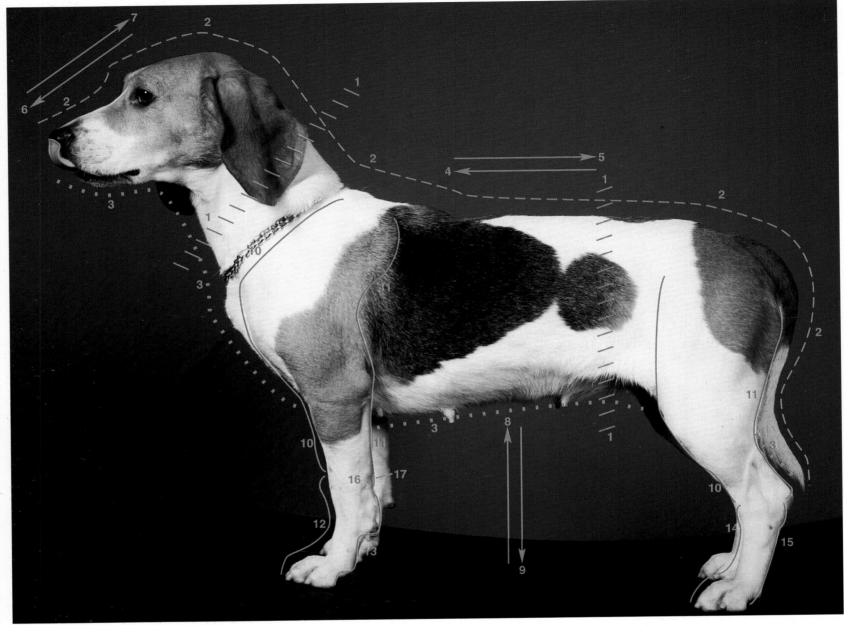

1 Lateral aspect of a standing live dog. The oblique dashes indicate the transverse plane, and the straight dashes, dots and continuous lines indicate the position and direction. Note, in particular, the specific terms for the head and the distal limbs.

1	Transverse plane of trunk	10	Cranial	} proximal limb
2	Dorsal } trunk and head	11	Caudal	
3	Ventral	12	Dorsal	} thoracic limb
4	Cranial } trunk	13	Palmar	(distal to carpus)
5	Caudal	14	Dorsal	} pelvic limb
6	Rostral } head	15	Plantar	(distal to tarsus)
7	Caudal	16	Lateral	} limb
8	Proximal } limb	17	Medial	
9	Distal			

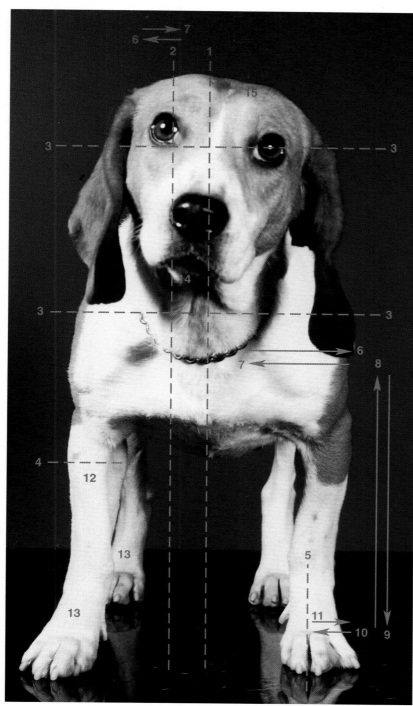

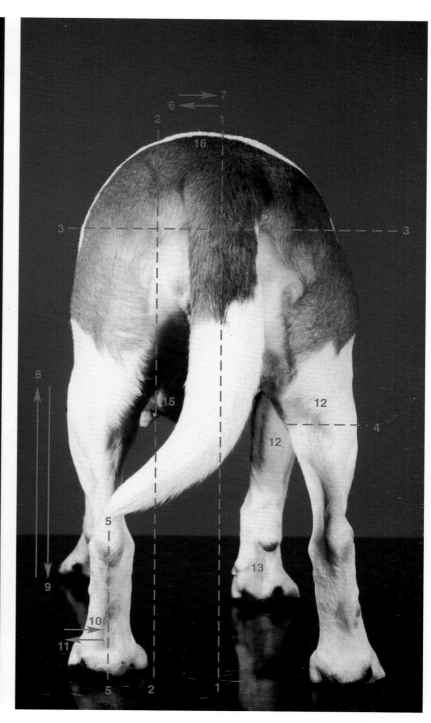

2 Cranial aspect of a standing live dog. The dotted lines indicate the anatomical planes of the body, and the arrows indicate the position and direction. Aspects of the head, trunk and limbs are marked by separate numbers.

3 Caudal aspect of a standing live dog. The dotted lines indicate the anatomical planes of the body, and the arrows indicate the position and direction. Aspects of the trunk and limbs are marked by separate numbers.

1	Median plane	8	Proximal ⎫
2	Sagittal plane	9	Distal ⎬ limb
3	Dorsal plane	10	Axial
4	Transverse	11	Abaxial
	plane ⎫ of limb	12	Cranial ⎫ limb
5	Axial plane ⎭	13	Dorsal ⎭
6	Lateral	14	Ventral ⎫ trunk and
7	Medial	15	Dorsal ⎭ head

● Note that the term para-median is sometimes applied to a sagittal plane that is close to the median plane.

1	Median plane	9	Distal ⎫
2	Sagittal plane	10	Axial
3	Dorsal plane	11	Abaxial ⎬ limbs
4	Transverse plane ⎫ of limb	12	Caudal
5	Axial plane ⎭	13	Palmar ⎭
6	Lateral ⎫ limb	14	Plantar
7	Medial ⎬	15	Ventral ⎫ trunk
8	Proximal ⎭	16	Dorsal ⎭

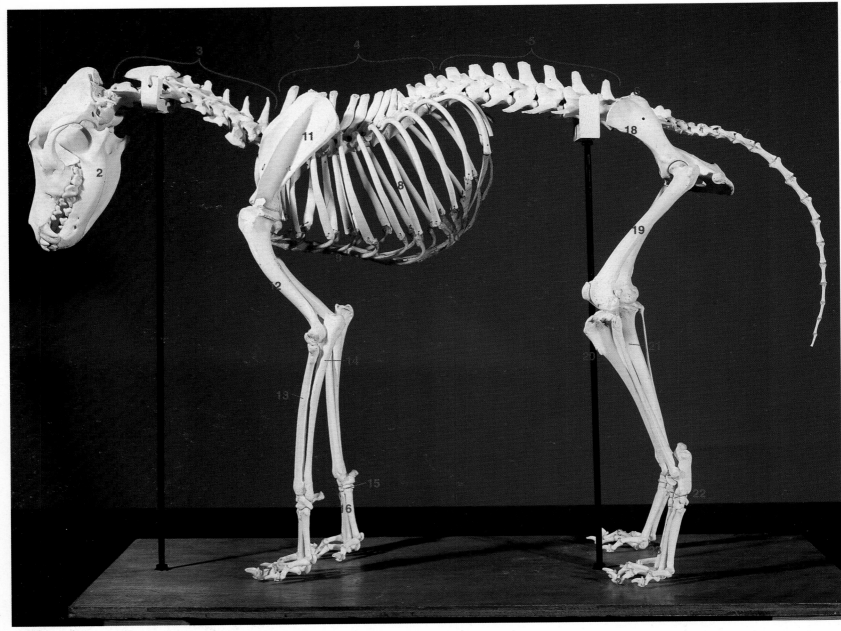

4 Lateral aspect of an articulated standing skeleton of a dog.

1	Skull	9	Sternum	17	Phalanges
2	Mandible	10	Costal arch	18	Ossa coxae
3	Cervical vertebrae	11	Scapula	19	Femur
4	Thoracic vertebrae	12	Humerus	20	Tibia
5	Lumbar vertebrae	13	Radius	21	Fibula
6	Sacrum	14	Ulna	22	Tarsus
7	Caudal vertebrae	15	Carpus	23	Metatarsus
8	Ribs	16	Metacarpus	24	Phalanges

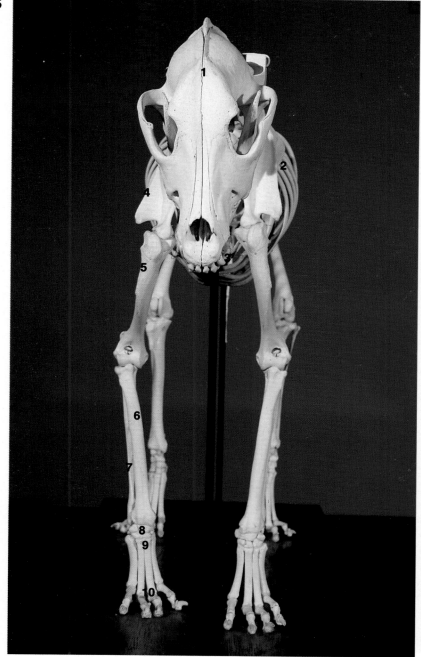

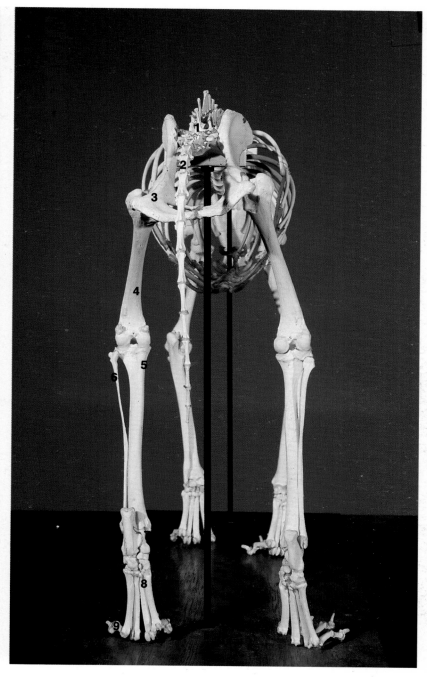

5 Cranial aspect of an articulated standing skeleton of a dog.

1	Skull	6	Radius
2	Ribs	7	Ulna
3	Sternum	8	Carpus
4	Scapula	9	Metacarpus
5	Humerus	10	Phalanges of manus

6 Caudal aspect of an articulated standing skeleton of a dog.

1	Sacrum	6	Fibula
2	Caudal vertebrae	7	Tarsus
3	Ossa coxae	8	Metatarsus
4	Femur	9	Phalanges of pes
5	Tibia		

2 Head and neck

Dealing with the structures of the head and neck, this chapter uses the live animal to indicate the palpable landmarks of the region, while the osteological features are demonstrated using bony specimens and radiographs. Soft tissue structures are illustrated in detail, with a series of prepared dissections, and their topographical relationships are displayed by means of additional cross-sectional specimens and radiography.

7 Lateral aspect of the head and neck region of a live dog, demonstrating palpable landmarks.

1	Incisive bone
2	Infraorbital foramen
3	Medial commissure of eyelids
4	Puncta lacrimale of upper lid (palpebra superior)
5	Puncta lacrimale of lower lid (palpebra inferior)
6	Third eyelid
7	Angular vein of the eye
8	Lateral commissure of eyelids
9	Maxilla
10	Zygomatic process of frontal bone
11	M. temporalis
12	Temporal line
13	External sagittal crest
14	External occipital protuberance
15	Pinna of ear
16	Zygomatic arch
17	M. masseter
18	Angular process of mandible
19	Position of mandibular lymph nodes
20	Body of mandible
21	Commissure of lips
22	Tongue (extruded)
23	Larynx
24	External jugular (site for venipuncture)

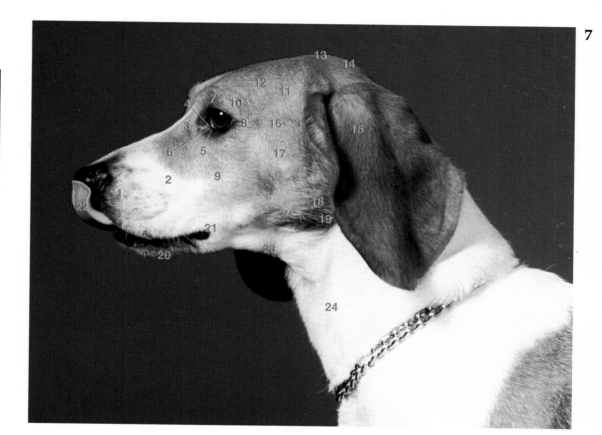

7

8 Cranial aspect of the head and neck region of a live dog, demonstrating palpable landmarks.

1	Planum nasale
2	Nares (nostril)
3	Philtrum
4	Upper lip (labia superior)
5	Tactile hairs
6	Incisive bone
7	Body of mandible
8	Nasal bones
9	Maxilla
10	Infraorbital foramen
11	Medial commissure of eyelids
12	Third eyelid
13	Lateral commissure of eyelid
14	Zygomatic arch
15	Zygomatic process of frontal bone
16	Frontal bone
17	M. temporalis
18	M. masseter
19	Pinna of ear

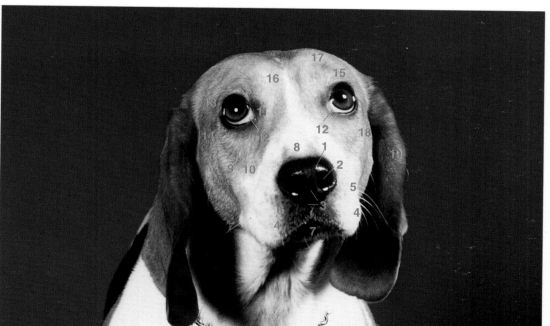

8

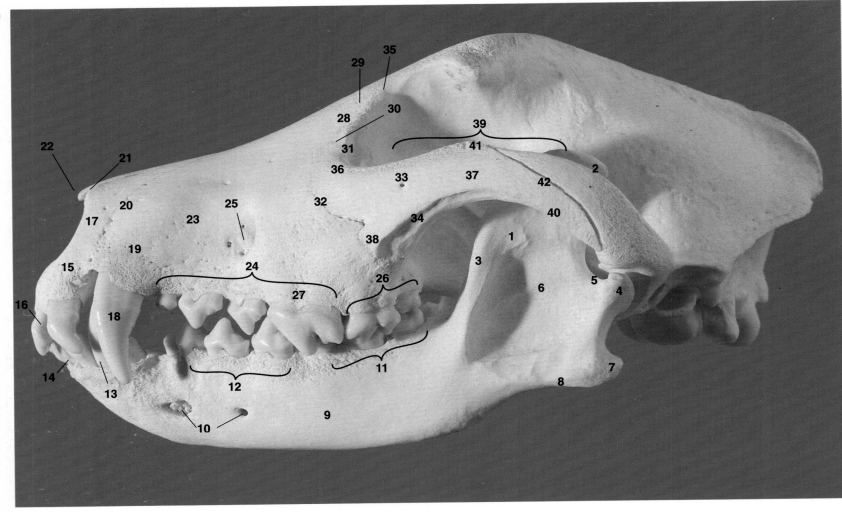

9   Lateral aspect of the skull and mandible of a bull terrier dog.

1	Ramus of mandible	15	Incisive bone	29	Frontomaxillary suture
2	Coronoid process	16	Upper incisor teeth	30	Lacrimomaxillary suture
3	Coronoid crest	17	Nasal process	31	Lacrimal bone
4	Condyloid process	18	Upper canine tooth	32	Zygomaticomaxillary suture
5	Mandibular notch	19	Alveolus of canine tooth	33	Infraorbital margin
6	Masseteric fossa	20	Incisivomaxillary suture	34	Masseteric margin
7	Angular process	21	Nasoincisive suture	35	Groove for angular vein of eye
8	Masseteric line	22	Nasal bone	36	Lacrimozygomatic suture
9	Body of mandible	23	Maxilla	37	Zygomatic bone
10	Mental foramina	24	Upper premolar teeth	38	Maxillary process
11	Lower molar teeth	25	Infraorbital foramen	39	Zygomatic arch
12	Lower premolar teeth	26	Upper molar teeth	40	Temporal process
13	Lower canine tooth	27	Alveolar juga	41	Frontal process
14	Lower incisor teeth	28	Frontal process	42	Temporozygomatic suture

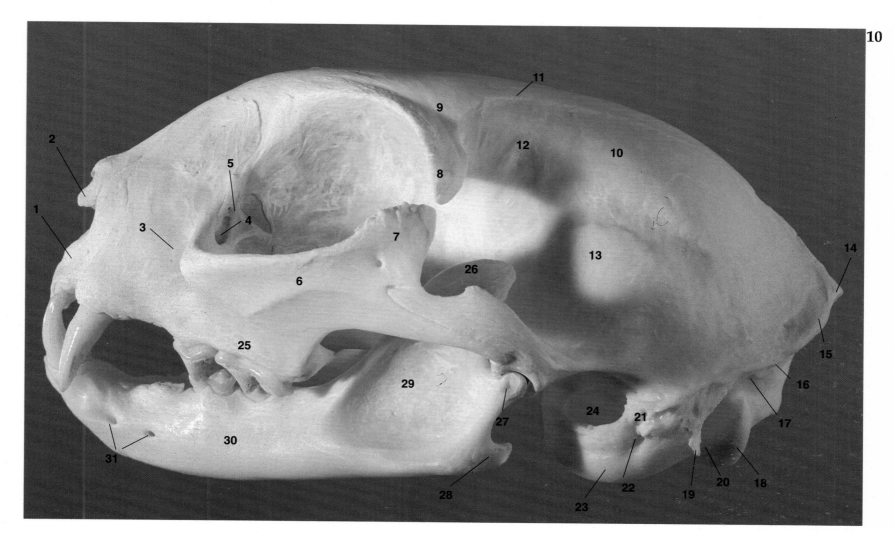

10 Lateral aspect of the skull and mandible of a cat.

1	Incisive bone	12	Temporal fossa	23	Tympanic bulla
2	Nasal bone	13	Squamous temporal bone	24	External acoustic meatus
3	Infraorbital foramen	14	External occipital protuberance	25	Maxilla
4	Fossa for lacrimal sac	15	Nuchal crest	26	Coronoid process
5	Lacrimal bone	16	Occipital bone	27	Condyloid process
6	Zygomatic bone	17	Dorsal condyloid fossa	28	Angular process
7	Frontal process of zygomatic bone	18	Occipital condyle	29	Masseteric fossa
8	Zygomatic process of frontal bone	19	Jugular process	30	Body of mandible
9	Frontal bone	20	Ventral condyloid fossa	31	Mental foramina
10	Parietal bone	21	Mastoid process		
11	Temporal line	22	Stylomastoid foramen		

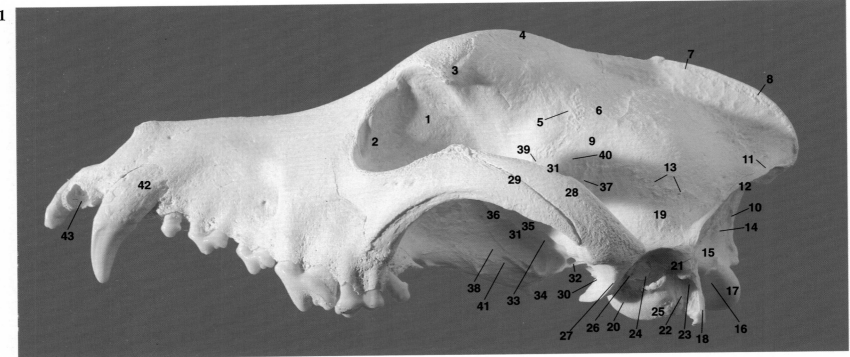

11 Lateral aspect of the skull of a dog, without the mandible.

1	Frontal bone	11	Occipitoparietal suture	23	Stylomastoid foramen	35	Orbital fissure
2	Fossa for lacrimal gland	12	Nuchal line	24	External acoustic meatus	36	Orbital canal
3	Zygomatic process of 1	13	Squamous suture	25	Tympanic bulla	37	Sphenosquamous suture
4	Temporal line	14	Mastoid foramen	26	Retroarticular foramen	38	Sphenopalatine suture
5	Frontoparietal suture (coronal suture)	15	Dorsal condyloid fossa	27	Retroarticular process	39	Sphenofrontal suture
		16	Ventral condyloid fossa	28	Zygomatic process	40	Sphenoparietal suture
6	Parietal bone	17	Occipital condyle	29	Temporozygomatic suture	41	Pterygosphenoid suture
7	External sagittal crest	18	Jugular process	30	Mandibular fossa	42	Alveolus of canine tooth (lateral wall partially resected)
8	Interparietal process and parietointerparietal suture	19	Squamous } part of temporal	31	Sphenoid bone		
		20	Tympanic } bone	32	Caudal alar foramen	43	Alveolus of incisor tooth
9	Temporal fossa	21	Mastoid process	33	Rostral alar foramen		
10	Occipital bone	22	Tympano-occipital suture	34	Pterygoid bone		

12 Lateral aspect of the skull of a cat. The zygomatic arch has been removed from the left side.

1	Parietal bone
2	Squamous temporal bone
3	Wing of basisphenoid bone
4	Presphenoid bone
5	Palatine bone
6	Pterygoid bone
7	External acoustic meatus
8	Stylomastoid foramen
9	Ethmoid foramina
10	Optic canal
11	Orbital fissure
12	Rostral alar foramen
13	Caudal alar foramen
14	Sphenopalatine foramen
15	Maxilla
16	Incisive bone
17	Incisor teeth
18	Canine tooth
19	Premolar teeth
20	Molar tooth

13 Medial aspect of a sagittal section of the left half of the skull of a cat.

1	Parietal bone
2	Frontal bone
3	Frontal sinus
4	Ethmoturbinates
5	Cribriform plate
6	Ethmoidal foramina
7	Nasal bone
8	Dorsal nasal concha
9	Ventral nasal concha
10	Incisive bone
11	Maxilla
12	Vomer
13	Alveoli of third premolar and first molar
14	Sphenoidal sinus
15	Presphenoid bone
16	Basisphenoid bone
17	Optic canal
18	Dorsum sellae
19	Tentorium osseum
20	Internal acoustic meatus
21	Jugular foramen
22	Hypoglossal canal
23	Occipital bone

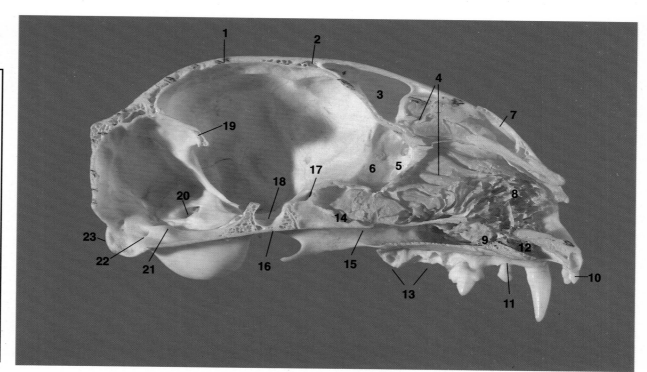

14 Dorsal aspect of the skull of a cat.

1	Incisive bone	9	Temporal bone
2	Nasal bone	10	Zygomatic process of temporal bone
3	Maxilla	11	Parietal bone
4	Frontal bone	12	Interparietal bone
5	Zygomatic process of frontal bone	13	Sagittal crest
6	Zygomatic bone	14	Occipital bone
7	Frontal process		
8	Coronoid process of mandible		

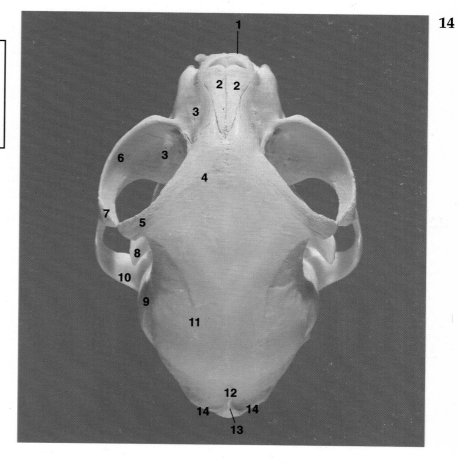

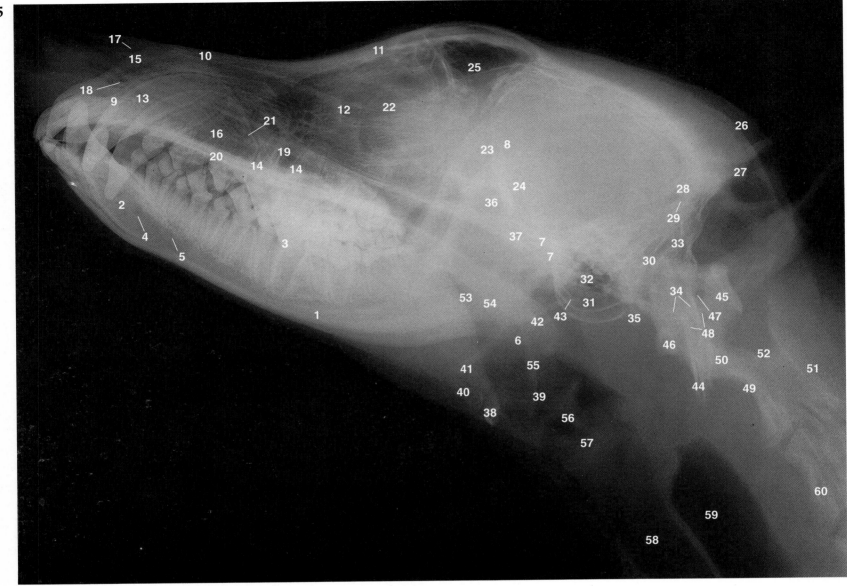

15 Lateral radiograph of the head of a dog.

1	Mandible	17	Dorsal nasal meatus	31	Tympanic bulla	46	Ventral arch
2	Lower canine	18	Ventral nasal meatus	32	External acoustic meatus	47	Intervertebral foramen
3	First lower molar	19	Maxillary sinus	33	Condyloid fossa	48	Transverse foramen
4	Mental foramina	20	Hard palate	34	Occipital condyle	49	Body {of second cervical vertebra
5	Mandibular canal	21	Infraorbital foramen	35	Jugular process		(axis)
6	Angular process	22	Orbit	36	Presphenoid bone	50	Dens (odontoid process)
7	Condyloid process	23	Temporal process of zygomatic	37	Pterygoid process	51	Spinous process
8	Coronoid process		bone	38	Basihyoid bone	52	Cranial vertebral notch
9	Incisive bone	24	Zygomatic process of temporal	39	Thyrohyoid bone	53	Root of tongue
10	Nasal bone		bone	40	Keratohyoid bone	54	Soft palate
11	Frontal bone	25	Frontal sinus	41	Epihyoid bone	55	Epiglottis
12	Maxilla	26	Sagittal crest	42	Stylohyoid bone	56	Thyroid cartilage
13	Upper canine	27	External occipital protuberance	43	Tympanohyoid cartilage	57	Cricoid cartilage
14	Fourth upper premolar	28	Tentorium cerebelli osseum	44	Transverse process of first cervical	58	Trachea
15	Dorsal nasal concha	29	Transverse canal		vertebra (atlas)	59	Oesophagus
16	Ventral nasal concha	30	Petrous temporal bone	45	Dorsal arch	60	Third cervical vertebra

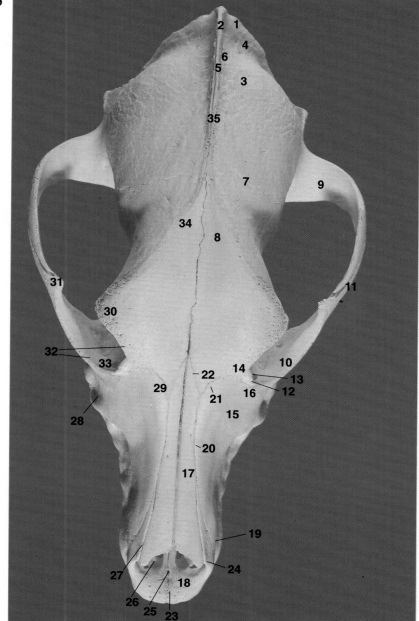

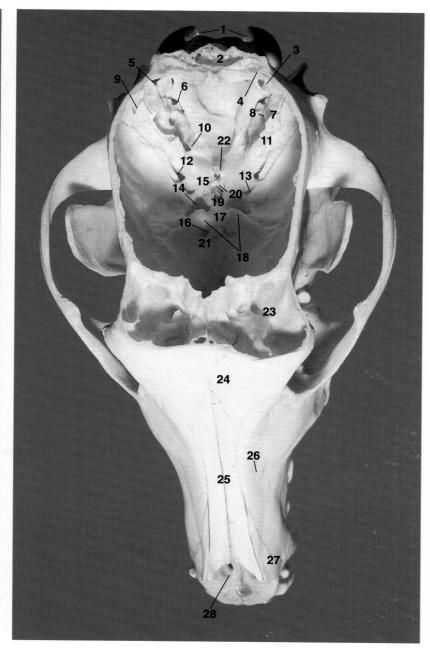

16 Dorsal aspect of the skull of a dog.

1	Occipital bone	19	Incisivomaxillary suture
2	Interparietal bone	20	Nasomaxillary suture
3	Parietal bone	21	Frontomaxillary suture
4	Occipitoparietal suture	22	Frontonasal suture
5	Sagittal suture	23	Interincisive suture
6	Parietointerparietal suture	24	Nasoincisive suture
7	Parietofrontal or coronal suture	25	Incisive canal
8	Frontal bone	26	Palatine fissure
9	Squamous part of temporal bone	27	Nasal process of 18
10	Zygomatic bone	28	Infraorbital foramen
11	Temporozygomatic bone	29	Frontal process of 15
12	Lacrimal bone	30	Zygomatic process of 8
13	Lacrimozygomatic suture		(supraorbital process)
14	Frontolacrimal suture	31	Frontal process of 10
15	Maxilla	32	Orbital margin
16	Lacrimomaxillary suture	33	Fossa for lacrimal sac
17	Nasal bone	34	Temporal line
18	Incisive bone	35	External sagittal crest

17 Dorsal aspect of the skull of a dog, with the dorsal calvaria removed.
The angulation reveals the caudal structures of the cranial vault.

1	Occipital bone	15	Presphenoid bone
2	Transverse canal	16	Optic canal
3	Condyloid canal	17	Sulcus chiasmatis
4	Hypoglossal canal	18	Rostral clinoid process
5	Mastoid foramen	19	Hypophyseal fossa
6	Jugular foramen	20	Caudal clinoid process
7	Cerebellar fossa	21	Basisphenoid bone
8	Internal acoustic meatus	22	Dorsum sellae
9	Canal for transverse sinus	23	Frontal sinus (lateral part)
10	Canal for trigeminal nerve	24	Frontal bone
11	Crista partis petrosae	25	Nasal bone
12	Foramen ovale	26	Maxilla
13	Foramen rotundum	27	Incisive bone
14	Orbital fissure	28	Palatine fissure

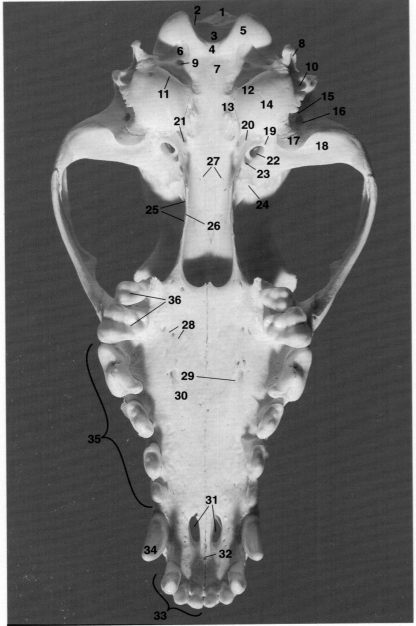

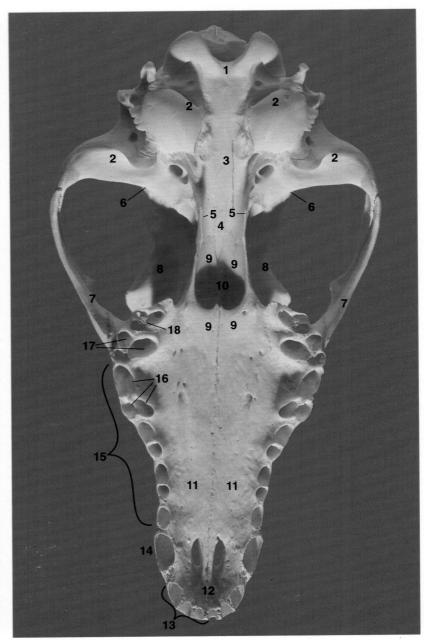

18 Ventral aspect of the skull of a dog, showing the upper dental arches.

1	External occipital protuberance	20	Foramen lacerum
2	Nuchal tubercle	21	Musculotubal canal
3	Foramen magnum	22	Foramen ovale with spinous foramen
4	Intercondyloid incisure	23	Caudal alar foramen
5	Condyloid process	24	Rostral alar foramen
6	Ventral condyloid fossa	25	Orbital fissure
7	Pharyngeal tubercle	26	Optic canal
8	Jugular process	27	Caudal foramen of pterygoid canal
9	Hypoglossal canal	28	Minor palatine foramen
10	Stylomastoid foramen	29	Major palatine foramen
11	Tympano-occipital fissure	30	Palatine sulcus
12	Jugular foramen	31	Palatine fissure
13	Muscular tubercle	32	Incisive canal
14	Tympanic bulla	33	Incisor teeth
15	External acoustic meatus	34	Canine tooth
16	Temporal meatus	35	Premolar teeth
17	Retroarticular process	36	Molar teeth
18	Mandibular fossa		
19	Petrotympanic fissure		

19 Ventral aspect of the skull of a dog. The upper teeth have been removed to reveal the alveolar pattern of the upper dental arch.

1	Occipital bone	10	Vomer
2	Temporal bone	11	Maxilla
3	Basisphenoid bone	12	Incisive bone
4	Presphenoid bone	13	Alveoli of incisor teeth
5	Pterygoid bone	14	Alveolus of canine tooth
6	Parietal bone	15	Alveoli of premolar teeth
7	Zygomatic bone	16	Alveolus of fourth premolar tooth
8	Frontal bone	17	Alveolus of first molar tooth
9	Palatine bone	18	Alveolus of second molar tooth

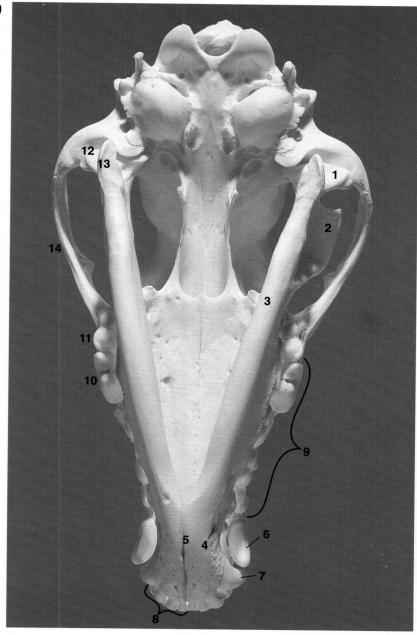

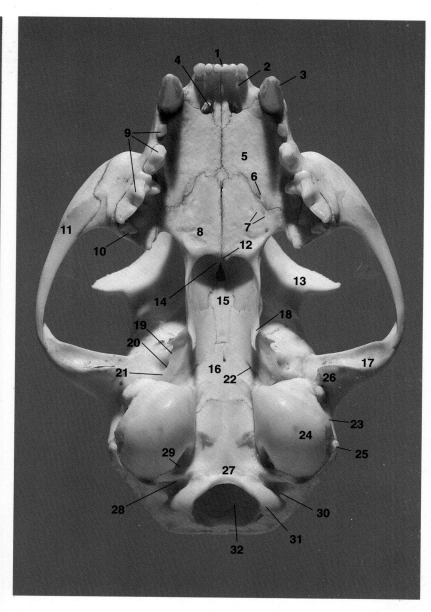

21 Ventral aspect of the skull of a cat. A marker dye has been used to highlight the suture lines.

20 Ventral aspect of the skull and mandible of a dog.

1	Condyloid process	8	Lower incisor tooth
2	Coronoid process	9	Upper premolar teeth
3	Body of mandible	10	Fourth upper premolar tooth
4	Mental foramina	11	First upper molar tooth
5	Mandibular symphysis	12	Temporomandibular joint
6	Upper canine tooth	13	Angular process
7	Lower canine tooth	14	Zygomatic arch

1	Incisor teeth	18	Hamulus of pterygoid
2	Incisive bone	19	Rostral alar foramen
3	Canine tooth	20	Caudal alar foramen
4	Palatine fissure	21	Foramen ovale
5	Maxilla	22	Pterygoid canal
6	Major palatine foramen	23	External acoustic meatus
7	Minor palatine foramina	24	Tympanic bulla
8	Palatine bone	25	Stylomastoid foramen
9	Premolar teeth	26	Retroarticular process
10	Molar tooth	27	Occipital bone
11	Zygomatic bone	28	Jugular process
12	Caudal nasal spine of 8	29	Jugular foramen
13	Frontal bone	30	Ventral condyloid fossa
14	Vomer	31	Occipital condyle (condyloid process)
15	Presphenoid bone		
16	Basisphenoid bone	32	Foramen magnum
17	Mandibular fossa		

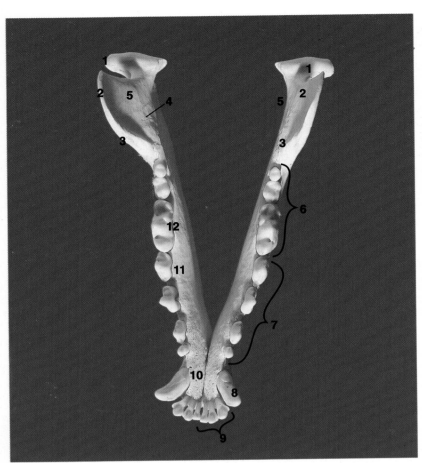

22 Dorsal aspect of the mandible of a dog.

1	Condyloid process
2	Coronoid process
3	Coronoid crest
4	Mandibular foramen
5	Ramus of mandible
6	Lower molar teeth
7	Lower premolar teeth
8	Lower canine tooth
9	Lower incisor teeth
10	Mandibular symphysis
11	Body of mandible
12	Mylohyoid crest

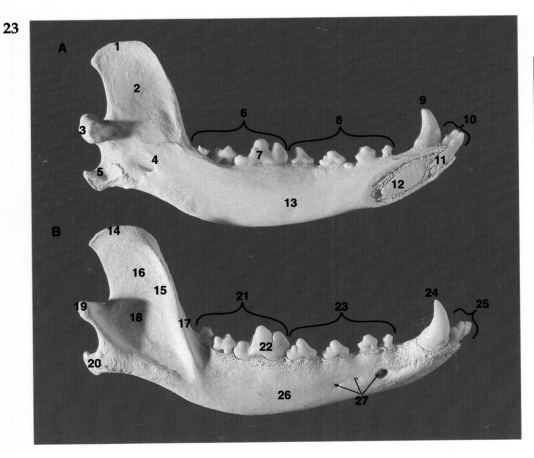

23 Medial (A) and lateral (B) aspect of the mandible of a dog.

1	Coronoid process
2	Ramus of mandible
3	Condyloid process
4	Mandibular foramen
5	Angular process
6	Molar teeth
7	First molar tooth
8	Premolar teeth
9	Canine tooth
10	Incisor teeth
11	Alveolus of incisor tooth
12	Canine root in alveolus
13	Body of mandible
14	Coronoid process
15	Coronoid crest
16	Ramus
17	Mandibular notch
18	Masseteric fossa
19	Condyloid process
20	Angular process
21	Molar teeth
22	First molar tooth
23	Premolar teeth
24	Canine tooth
25	Incisor teeth
26	Body of mandible
27	Mental foramina

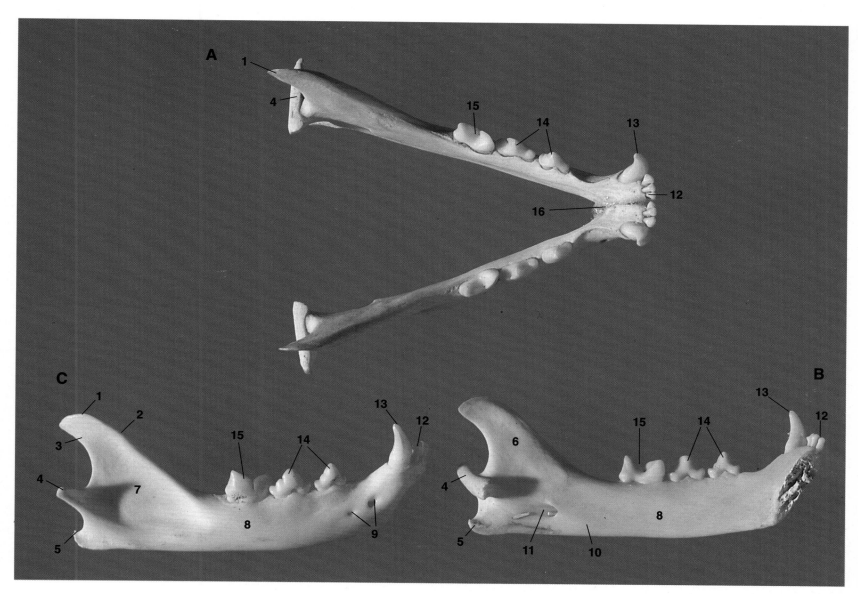

24 Dorsal aspect (A) of the left and right mandibles, medial aspect (B) of the left mandible and lateral aspect (C) of the right mandible of a cat.

1	Coronoid process	9	Mental foramina
2	Coronoid crest	10	Mylohyoid crest
3	Mandibular notch	11	Mandibular foramen
4	Condyloid process	12	Incisor teeth
5	Angular process	13	Canine tooth
6	Ramus of mandible	14	Premolar teeth
7	Masseteric fossa	15	Molar tooth
8	Body of mandible	16	Mandibular symphysis

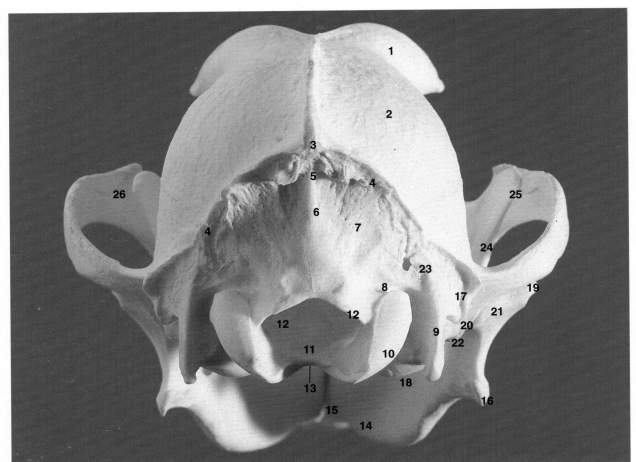

25 Caudal aspect of the skull and mandible of a dog.

1	Frontal bone
2	Parietal bone
3	Interparietal bone
4	Nuchal crest
5	External occipital protuberance
6	External occipital crest
7	Supraoccipital bone
8	Exoccipital bone
9	Jugular process
10	Occipital condyle
11	Foramen magnum
12	Nuchal tubercle
13	Intercondyloid notch
14	Body of mandible
15	Mandibular symphysis
16	Angular process
17	Temporal bone
18	Tympanic bulla
19	Zygomatic process
20	Mastoid process
21	Temporomandibular joint
22	Area of attachment of tympanohyoid
23	Mastoid foramen
24	Ramus of mandible
25	Coronoid process
26	Zygomatic bone

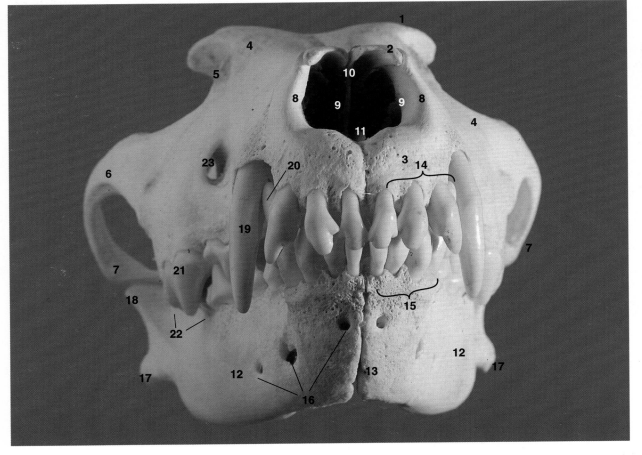

26 Rostral aspect of the skull and mandible of a dog.

1	Frontal bone
2	Nasal bone
3	Incisive bone
4	Maxilla
5	Lacrimal bone
6	Zygomatic bone
7	Zygomatic process of temporal bone
8	Osseous nasal opening
9	Nasal fossae
10	Nasal septum
11	Vomer
12	Body of mandible
13	Mandibular symphysis
14	Upper incisor teeth
15	Lower incisor teeth
16	Mental foramina
17	Angular process
18	Temporomandibular joint
19	Upper canine tooth
20	Lower canine tooth
21	Fourth upper premolar tooth
22	First lower molar tooth
23	Infraorbital foramen

27 Frontomandibular radiograph of the head of a dog.

1 Spinous process of second cervical vertebra (axis)
2 Dens (odontoid process)
3 Cranial articular surface
4 Transverse process of first cervical vertebral (atlas)
5 Alar notch
6 Transverse foramen
7 Caudal articular surface
8 Cranial articular surface
9 Nuchal line
10 Nuchal tubercle
11 Occipital condyle
12 Foramen magnum
13 Jugular process
14 Mastoid process
15 Petrous temporal bone
16 Crista partis petrosae
17 Tympanic bulla
18 External acoustic meatus
19 Hypophyseal fossa
20 Optic canal
21 Ethmoid fossa
22 Pterygoid process
23 Ethmoturbinates
24 Frontal sinus
25 Vomer
26 Palatine fissure
27 Medial wall of orbit
28 Zygomatic arch
29 Frontal process of zygomatic bone
30 Condyloid process
31 Angular process
32 Body of mandible
33 Coronoid process
34 Fourth upper premolar tooth
35 Upper canine tooth
36 Lower canine tooth

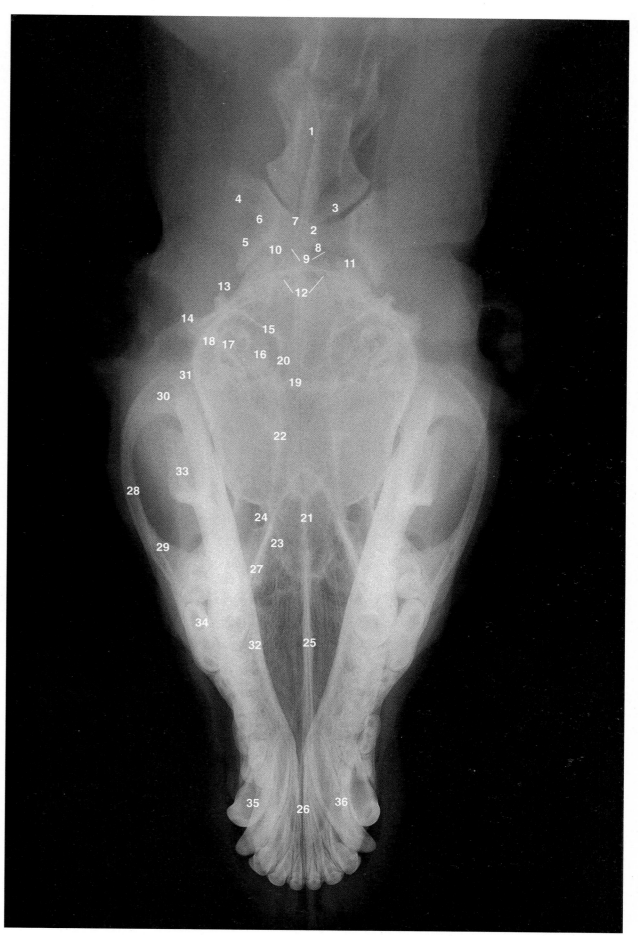

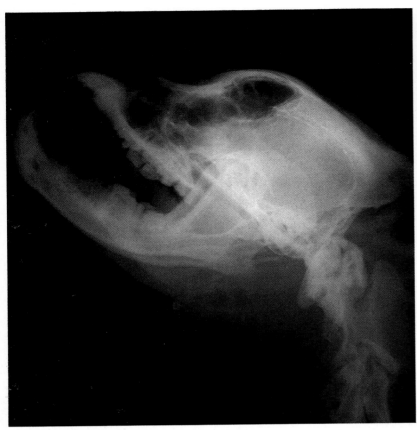

28 Lateral radiograph of the head of a brachycephalic breed of dog, demonstrating the greatly foreshortened facial portion of the skull.

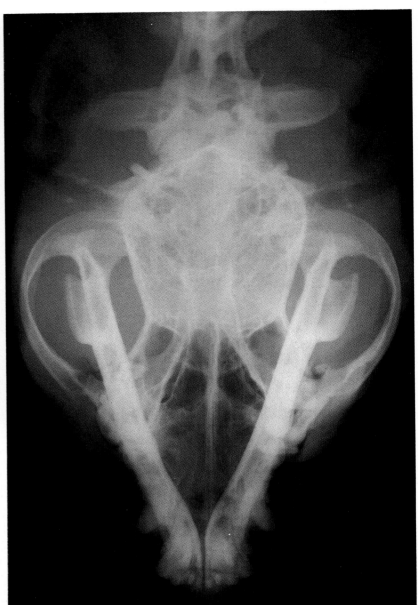

29 Mandibulofrontal radiograph of the head of a brachycephalic breed of dog, demonstrating the malocclusion of the upper and lower dental arches.

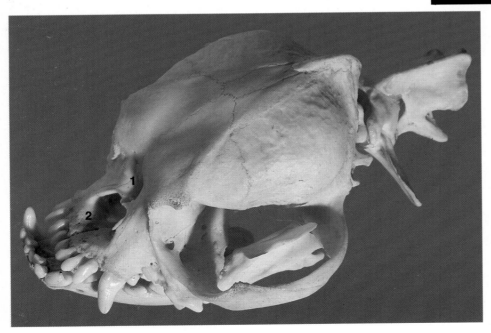

30 Dorsolateral aspect of the skull of a brachycephalic breed of dog, demonstrating the foreshortened facial region and the malocclusion of the dental arcade.

1	Frontal fossa
2	External nasal opening

31 Lateral aspect of a dolichocephalic skull of a dog, demonstrating the elongation of the facial region. There is an increased space between the canine and first premolar tooth (diastema).

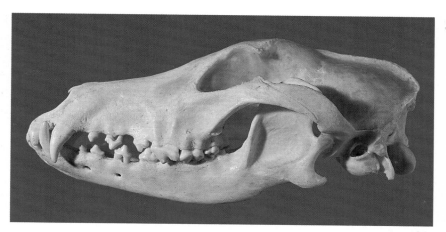

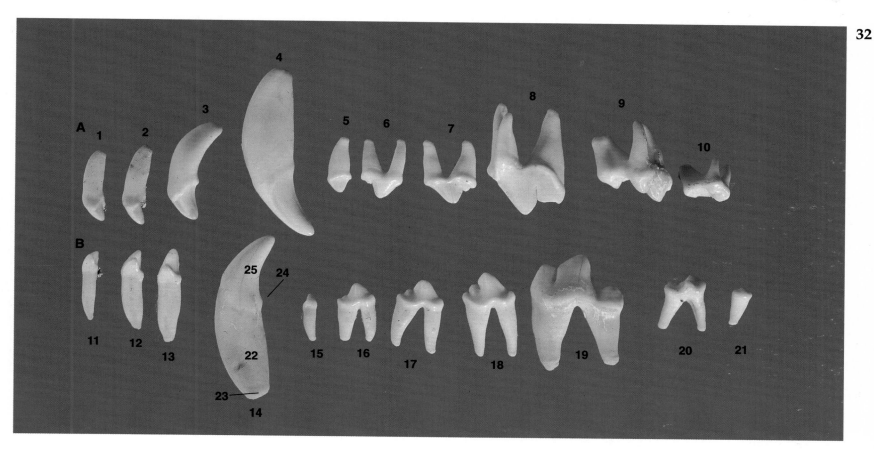

32 Dental arcade of an adult dog, showing the individual teeth from the upper (A) and lower (B) dental arch of the left half of a dog skull and mandible.

1	First	} upper incisor tooth	14	Lower canine tooth
2	Second		15	First
3	Third		16	Second } lower premolar tooth
4	Upper canine tooth		17	Third
5	First		18	Fourth
6	Second	upper premolar tooth	19	First
7	Third		20	Second } lower molar tooth
8	Fourth (carnassial)		21	Third
9	First	} upper molar tooth	22	Root covered in cementum
10	Second		23	Apex of root
11	First		24	Neck
12	Second	} lower incisor tooth	25	Crown covered in enamel
13	Third			

- Permanent dentition:
  $2 \{I \tfrac{3}{3} C \tfrac{1}{1} P \tfrac{4}{4} M \tfrac{2}{3}\} = 42$

- The upper fourth premolar and lower first molar are the carnassial or sectorial teeth.

- Deciduous dentition:
  $2 \{Di \tfrac{3}{3} Dc \tfrac{1}{1} Dp \tfrac{3}{3}\} = 28$

- The first premolar in both the upper and lower jaw appears with the deciduous dentition, but is not replaced and persists with the permanent dentition. Note the wide diameter of the root of the adult canine tooth, which makes it difficult to extract by simple traction, and also the trifid root system of the fourth upper premolar. This widespread root system necessitates the use of a dental elevator to loosen the tooth within the alveolus before extraction.

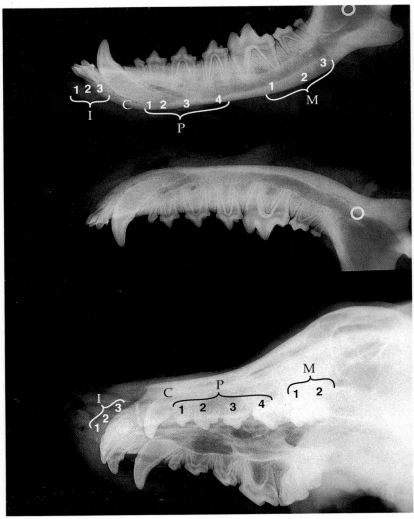

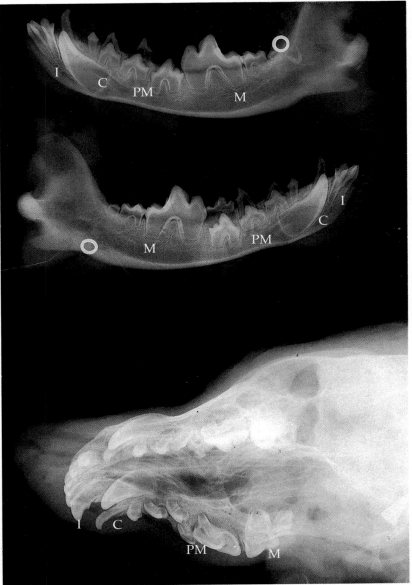

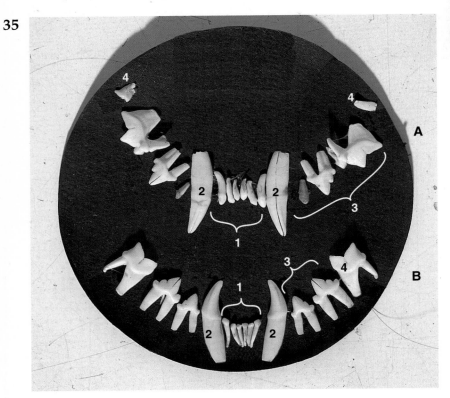

33 Radiograph of a disarticulated mandible with the two bodies separated, and an obliquely positioned skull, demonstrating the root formation of the adult canine dentition.

34 Radiograph of the disarticulated and divided mandible and the obliquely positioned skull of a puppy, demonstrating the replacement of the deciduous dentition by the permanent dental arches. The deciduous incisors have been lost and the deciduous canines and premolars can be seen above their permanent replacements. Note that the first premolar occurs in the deciduous arch, but remains as a permanent tooth.

35 Dental arcade of an adult cat, showing the individual teeth from the upper (A) and lower (B) dental arch.

1	Incisor teeth
2	Canine tooth
3	Premolar teeth
4	Molar tooth

- Permanent dentition:
  $2 \{ I \tfrac{3}{3} C \tfrac{1}{1} P \tfrac{3}{2} M \tfrac{1}{1} \} = 30$

- The third upper premolar and first lower molar are the sectorial teeth.
- Deciduous dentition:
  $2 \{ Di \tfrac{3}{3} Dc \tfrac{1}{1} Dp \tfrac{3}{2} \} = 26$

36 Lateral aspect of the head of a dog. Only the skin has been resected to reveal the superficial muscles.

1	M. platysma
2	M. sphincter colli superficialis
3	External jugular vein
4	M. parotidoauricularis
5	M. zygomaticoauricularis
6	M.m. cervicoauricularis
7	M. sphincter colli profundus
8	M. zygomaticus
9	M. orbicularis oris
10	M. levator nasolabialis
11	M. frontalis
12	M. orbicularis oculi
13	M. retractor anguli oculi lateralis
14	M. scutuloauricularis
15	Palpebral nerve (VII)
16	Zygomaticotemporal nerve (V)

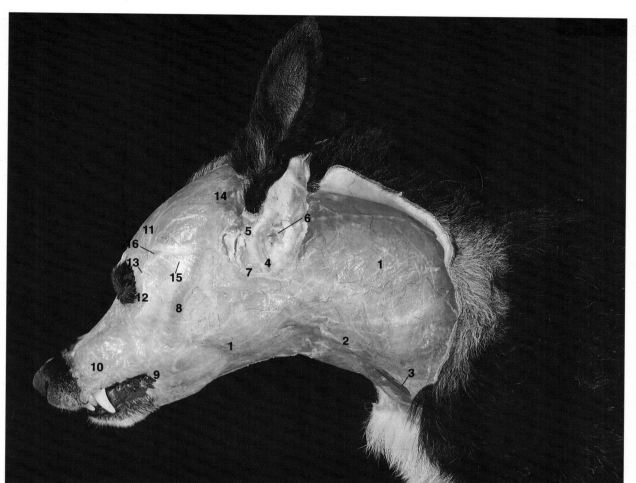

37 Lateral aspect of the head of a dog after removal of the superficial muscles.

1	M. sternomastoideus
2	M. sterno-occipitalis
3	M. cleidocervicalis
4	External jugular vein
5	Mandibular salivary gland
6	Mandibular lymph node
7	M. digastricus
8	M. parotidoauricularis
9	Linguofacial vein
10	M. mylohyoideus
11	Maxillary vein
12	Parotid salivary gland
13	M. masseter
14	Parotid duct
15	Facial vein
16	M. buccinator
17	Lingual vein
18	M. orbicularis oris
19	M. levator nasolabialis
20	M. levator labii maxillaris
21	M. zygomaticus
22	M. frontalis
23	M. retractor anguli oculi lateralis
24	M. temporalis
25	Zygomatic arch
26	Zygomaticotemporal nerve (V)
27	Palpebral nerve (VII)
28	Dorsal buccal branch (VII)
29	Ventral buccal branch (VII)
30	Auriculotemporal nerve (V)

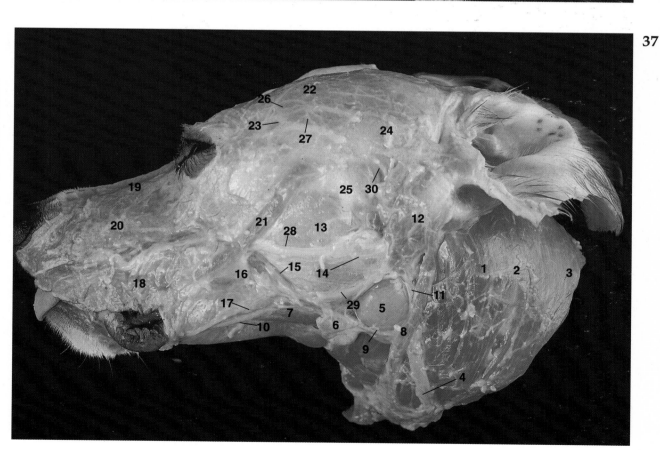

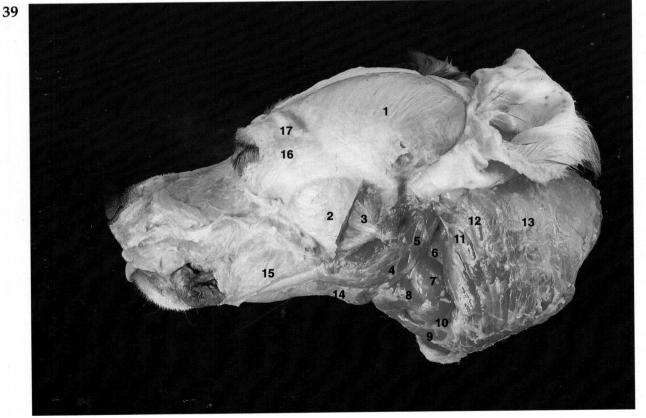

38 Dorsal aspect of the superficial muscles of the head of a dog.

1 M. cervicoscutularis	9 M. retractor anguli oculi lateralis
2 M. cervicoauricularis	10 M. levator anguli oculi medialis
3 Cutaneous branch of second cervical nerve	11 M. levator nasolabialis
4 M. interscutularis	12 Planum nasale
5 M. frontalis (cut edge)	13 Palpebral rim
6 M. scutuloauricularis (cut edge)	14 Palpebral nerve (VII)
7 M. zygomaticus	15 Branches of rostral auricular nerve (VII)
8 M. orbicularis occuli	16 M. temporalis

39 Lateral aspect of the muscles of the head of a dog after removal of the skin and cutaneous muscles.

1 M. temporalis	
2 Superficial ⎱ part of	
3 Middle ⎰ M. masseter	
4 M. digastricus	
5 M. stylohyoideus	
6 Retropharyngeal lymph node	
7 M. thyropharyngeus	
8 M. thyrohyoideus	
9 M. sternohyoideus	
10 M. sternothyroideus	
11 M. sternomastoideus ⎱ M. sterno-	
12 M. sterno-occipitalis ⎰ cephalicus	
13 M. cleidocervicalis	
14 M. mylohyoideus	
15 M. buccinator	
16 M. retractor anguli oculi lateralis	
17 M. frontalis (cut edge)	

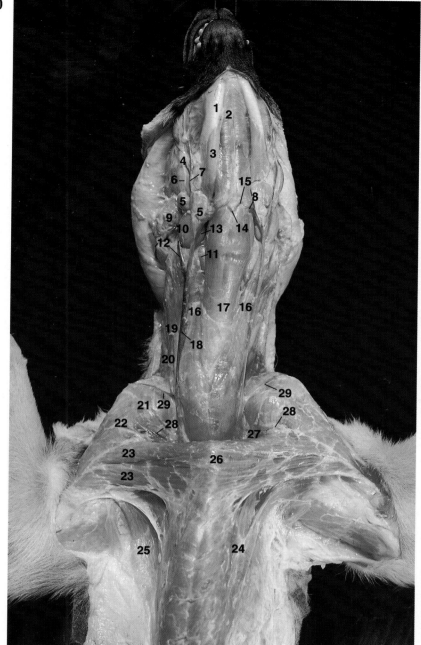

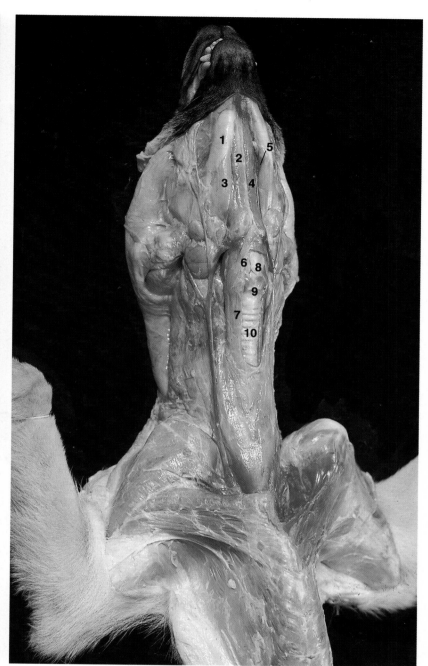

40 Ventral aspect of the superficial muscles of the head and neck of a dog.

41 Ventral aspect of the head and neck of a dog. The sternohyoideus and sternothyroideus muscles have been resected to expose the trachea.

1	Body of mandible	12	Maxillary vein	21	Clavicular tendon
2	M. mylohyoideus	13	Lingual vein	22	M. cleidobrachialis
3	M. digastricus	14	Hyoid venous arch		(M. brachio-
4	M. masseter	15	Submental vein		cephalicus)
5	Mandibular lymph	16	M. sterno-	23	Mm. pectorales
	nodes		mastoideus and M.		superficiales
6	Parotid duct		sterno-occipitalis	24	M. pectoralis
7	Facial vein		(M. sterno-		profundus
8	M. stylohyoideus		cephalicus)	25	M. latissimus dorsi
9	Parotid gland	17	M. sternohyoideus	26	Manubrium sterni
10	Mandibular salivary	18	External jugular	27	Supraclavicular
	gland		vein		fossa
11	Medial	19	M. cleido-	28	Cephalic vein
	retropharyngeal		mastoideus	29	Omobrachial vein
	lymph node	20	M. cleidocervicalis		

1	Body of mandible	6	M. thyrohyoideus
2	M. mylohyoideus	7	M. sternothyroideus
3	M. digastricus	8	Thyroid cartilage
4	M. geniohyoideus	9	Cricoid cartilage
5	M. styloglossus	10	Trachea

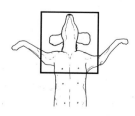

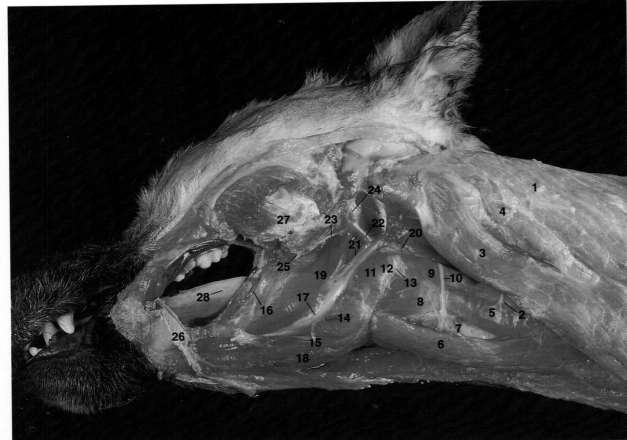

42 Ventrolateral aspect of the muscles of the head and neck of a dog. The left ramus and body of the mandible have been removed by sectioning off the muscles close to their insertions on these structures.

1	M. cleidocervicalis
2	Second cervical nerve
3	M. sternomastoideus } M. sterno-
4	M. sterno-occipitalis } cephalicus
5	M. sternothyroideus
6	M. sternohyoideus
7	M. cricothyroideus
8	M. thyrohyoideus
9	M. thyropharyngeus
10	Cervical nerve
11	M. ceratopharyngeus
12	M. chondropharyngeus
13	Cranial laryngeal nerve
14	M. hyoglossus
15	M. geniohyoideus
16	Buccal nerve
17	Hypoglossal nerve
18	M. mylohyoideus
19	M. styloglossus
20	Vagosympathetic trunk
21	Lingual artery
22	External carotid artery
23	Facial artery
24	Maxillary artery
25	Lingual nerve (cut ends)
26	Body of mandible (cut)
27	M. masseter
28	Tongue (folliate papillae)

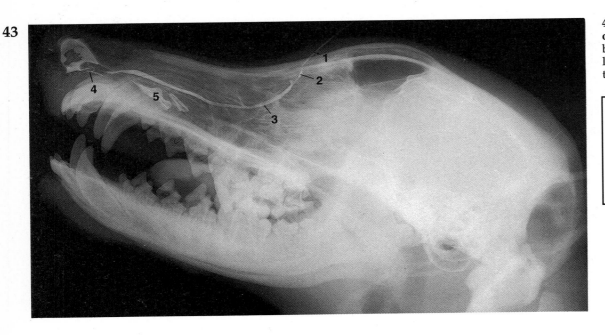

43 Lateral radiograph of the head of a dog. Radio-opaque material has been injected into the ventral lacrimal punctum to demonstrate the course of the nasolacrimal duct.

1	Needle in ventral lacrimal punctum
2	Lacrimal sac
3	Nasolacrimal duct
4	Duct discharging into floor of nasal vestibule
5	Refluxed radio-opaque material in ventral meatus

44 Rostral aspect of a transverse section of the skull of a dog, at the level of the fourth upper premolar tooth.

1	Ethmoid bone	7	Vomer
2	Labyrinth (conchae)	8	Choana leading to
3	Perpendicular plate or lamina		nasopharyngeal meatus
4	Lateral lamina	9	Infraorbital canal
5	Maxillary recess	10	Nasolacrimal canal
6	Transverse lamina		

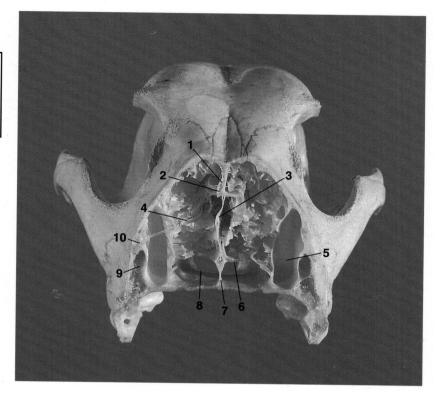

45 Transverse sections through the nasal cavity of a dog, at the level of (A) the upper canine tooth and (B) the fourth upper premolar tooth.

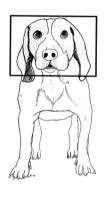

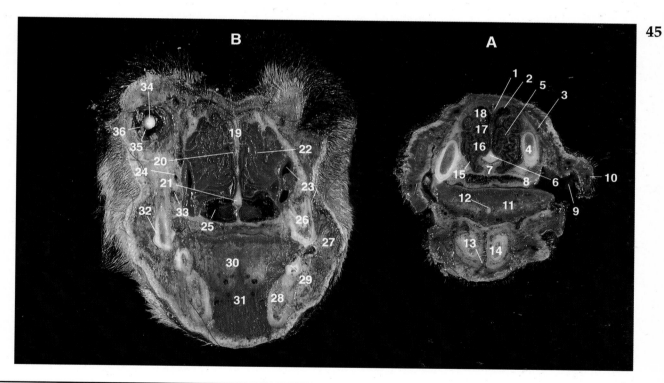

1	Nasal bone	11	Tongue	21	Vomer	31	M. geniohyoideus
2	Dorsal nasal concha	12	Lyssa	22	Ethmoidal conchae	32	Root canal of upper molar tooth
3	Maxilla	13	Body of mandible	23	Maxillary recess	33	Infraorbital canal
4	Upper canine tooth	14	Lower canine tooth	24	Nasolacrimal duct	34	Lens
5	Ventral nasal concha	15	Ventral meatus	25	Nasopharynx	35	Iris
6	Cartilaginous nasal septum	16	Common meatus	26	Fourth premolar tooth	36	Pupil
7	Vomer	17	Middle meatus	27	M. buccinator		
8	Hard palate	18	Dorsal meatus	28	Body of mandible		
9	Buccal cavity	19	Septal process of frontal bones	29	Lower premolar tooth		
10	Upper lip (labia superior)	20	Perpendicular plate, ethmoid bone	30	Tongue		

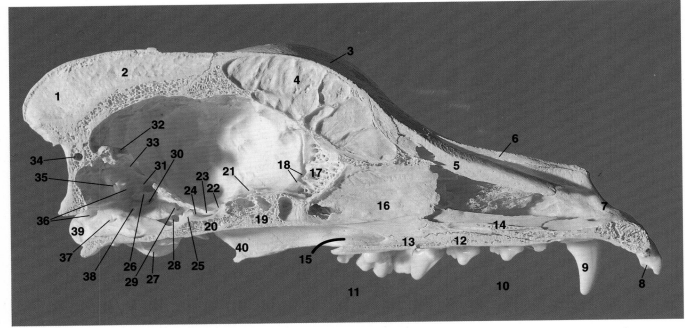

46 Median section of the skull of a dog.

1	Interparietal bone	13	Horizontal plate of palatine bone	21	Optical canal
2	Parietal bone			22	Orbital fissure
3	Frontal bone	14	Vomer	23	Foramen rotundum viewed through rostral alar foramen
4	Median septum of frontal sinus	15	Nasopharyngeal meatus		
		16	Osseous nasal septum of ethmoid bone	24	Foramen ovale
5	Nasal bone			25	Dorsum sellae
6	Maxilla	17	Cribriform plate of ethmoid bone with cribriform foramina	26	Petrosal ⎱ part of
7	Incisive bone			27	Tympanic ⎰ temporal bone
8	Incisor teeth			28	Internal carotid foramen
9	Canine tooth	18	Ethmoidal foramina	29	Canal for the trigeminal nerve
10	Premolar teeth	19	Body of presphenoid bone		
11	Molar teeth	20	Body of basisphenoid bone	30	Internal acoustic meatus
12	Palatine process of maxilla				

31	Cerebellar fossa
32	Tentorium osseum
33	Transverse groove
34	Transverse canal
35	Supramastoid foramen
36	Condyloid canal
37	Hypoglossal canal
38	Jugular foramen
39	Occipital bone
40	Pterygoid bone

47 Paramedian section of the skull of a dog.

1	Interparietal bone
2	Parietal bone
3	Frontal bone
4	Frontal sinus
5	Ectoturbinates (i–iii)
6	Cribriform plate
7	Ethmoidal foramina
8	Dorsal lamina
9	Endoturbinates (i–iv)
10	Nasal bone
11	Incisive bone
12	Dorsal nasal conchae
13	Ventral nasal conchae
14	Entrance to maxillary recess
15	Sphenopalatine foramen
16	Palatine process of maxilla
17	Horizontal plate of palatine bone
18	Nasopharyngeal meatus
19	Body of presphenoid bone
20	Body of basisphenoid bone
21	Pterygoid bone
22	Petrosal ⎱ part of
23	Tympanic ⎰ temporal bone
24	Occipital bone

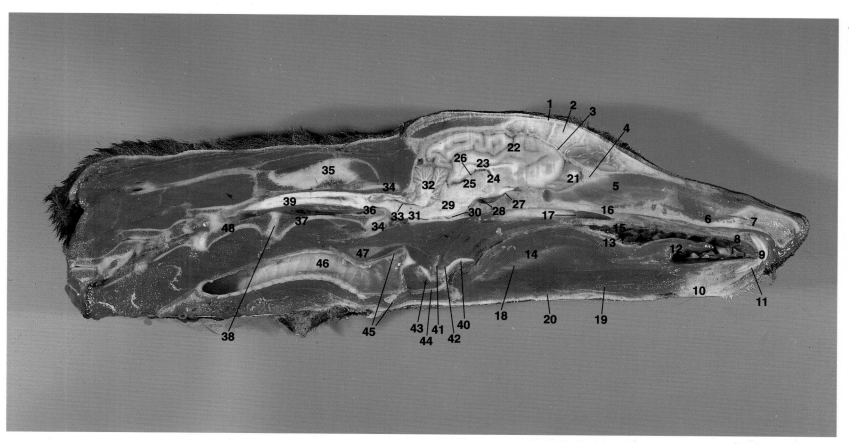

48   Median section of the head and neck of a dog, showing the left half of this region.

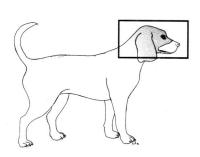

1	Frontal bone	26	Thalamus
2	Frontal sinus	27	Optic chiasma
3	Median septum	28	Site of hypophysis cerebri
4	Ethmoid bone	29	Pons
5	Osseous nasal septum	30	Transverse fibres of 29
6	Membranous septum	31	Medulla oblongata
7	Cartilaginous septum	32	Cerebellum
8	Incisive bone	33	Fourth ventricle
9	Upper incisor tooth	34	First cervical vertebra (atlas)
10	Mandible	35	Spinous process } of second cervical
11	Lower incisor tooth	36	Dens (odontoid process) } vertebra (axis)
12	Apex }	37	Body of axis
13	Dorsum } of tongue	38	Intervertebral disc with annulus fibrosus and inner
14	Body }		nucleus pulposus
15	Hard palate }	39	Spinal cord
16	Vomer	40	Epiglottis
17	Choana	41	Arytenoid cartilage
18	M. genioglossus	42	Aditus laryngis
19	M. geniohyoideus	43	Site of lateral ventricle
20	M. mylohyoideus	44	Thyroid cartilage
21	Olfactory bulb	45	Cricoid cartilage
22	Cerebral hemisphere	46	Trachea
23	Corpus callosum	47	Oesophagus
24	Third ventricle	48	Third cervical vertebra
25	Interthalamic adhesion		

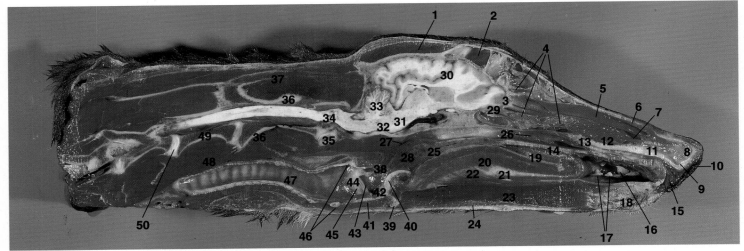

49

49 Paramedian section of the head and neck of a dog.

1	M. temporalis	18	Mandible	35	First cervical vertebra (atlas)
2	Frontal sinus	19	Apex (reflected caudally)	36	Second cervical vertebra (axis)
3	Cribriform plate of ethmoid bone	20	Body	37	M. rectus capitis dorsalis
4	Ethmoidal conchae	21	Lyssa	38	Laryngopharynx
5	Dorsal nasal concha	22	M. genioglossus	39	Hyoid bone
6	Dorsal meatus	23	M. geniohyoideus	40	Epiglottis
7	Middle meatus	24	M. mylohyoideus	41	Thyroid cartilage
8	Alar fold	25	Soft palate	42	Vestibular fold
9	Cartilage of nasal septum	26	Choana	43	Lateral ventricle
10	External nares (nostrils)	27	Opening of auditory tube	44	Vocal process of arytenoid cartilage
11	Ventral meatus	28	Nasopharynx	45	Vocal fold
12	Ventral nasal concha	29	Olfactory bulb	46	Cricoid cartilage
13	Vomer	30	Cerebral hemisphere	47	Trachea
14	Hard palate	31	Pons	48	M. longus colli
15	Upper lip (labia superior)	32	Medulla oblongata	49	Body of third cervical vertebra
16	Canine teeth	33	Cerebellum	50	Intervertebral disc with outer annulus fibrosus and inner nucleus pulposus
17	Premolar teeth	34	Spinal cord		

(19, 20 labelled "of tongue")

50

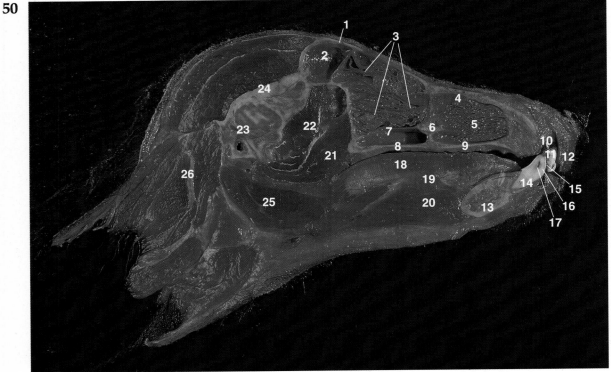

50 Paramedian section of the head of a dog, revealing the structures of the right nasal cavity.

1	Frontal bone
2	Lateral part of frontal sinus
3	Ethmoidal conchae
4	Dorsal nasal conchae
5	Ventral nasal conchae
6	Lateral lamina of ethmoid bone
7	Choana
8	Palatine bone
9	Maxilla
10	Incisive bone
11	Upper incisor tooth
12	Upper lip (labia superior)
13	Mandible
14	Lower canine tooth
15	Enamel
16	Dentine
17	Pulp cavity
18	Body of tongue
19	M. genioglossus
20	M. geniohyoideus
21	M. pterygoideus medialis
22	M. temporalis
23	Temporal bone
24	Parietal bone
25	M. digastricus
26	M. rectus capitis dorsalis

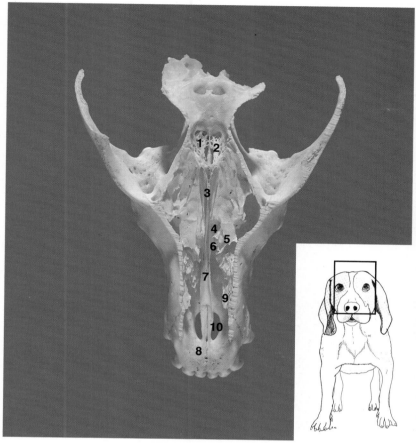

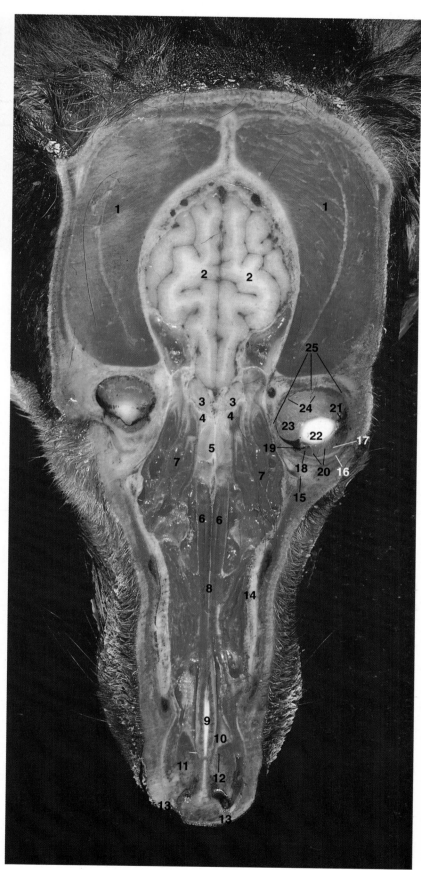

51 Nasal region of the skull of a dog, sectioned in the dorsal plane.

1	Ethmoid bone	6	Horizontal	} part of vomer
2	Cribriform plate	7	Sagittal	
3	Perpendicular plate or lamina	8	Incisive bone	
4	Transverse lamina	9	Ventral nasal conchae	
5	Endoturbinates	10	Palatine fissure	

52 Dorsal aspect of a coronal section through the head of a dog, at the level of the bony orbit, revealing the contents of the nasal cavity. The section has been made in the dorsal plane.

1	M. temporalis	14	Maxilla
2	Cerebral hemispheres	15	Lacrimal sac
3	Olfactory bulbs	16	Cornea
4	Cribriform plate ⎫ of ethmoid	17	Anterior chamber
5	Perpendicular plate ⎬ bone	18	Iris
6	Dorsal nasal conchae	19	Posterior chamber
7	Ethmoidal conchae	20	Pupil
8	Median septum	21	Ciliary body
9	Cartilaginous septum	22	Lens
10	Alar fold	23	Vitreous chamber
11	Nasal vestibule	24	Fundus
12	Opening of nasolacrimal duct	25	Orbit
13	Nares (nostrils)		

53

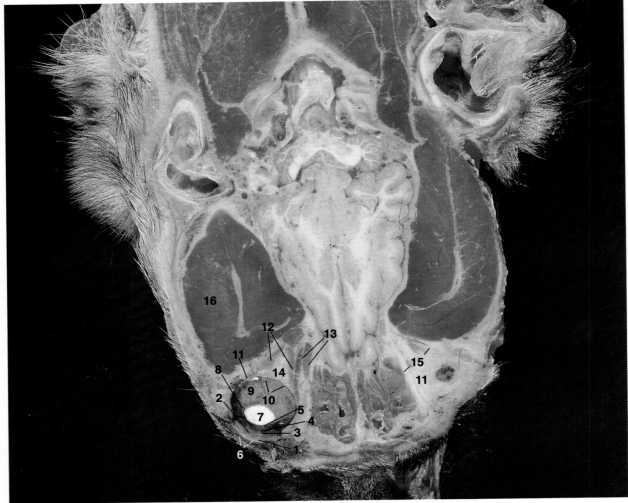

53 Dorsal aspect of an oblique section in the dorsal plane, made through the head of a dog at the level of the orbit. The structure of the eyeball and the orbital contents are shown.

1	Bulbar conjunctiva covering cornea
2	Cornea
3	Anterior chamber
4	Iris
5	Posterior chamber
6	Pupil
7	Lens
8	Ciliary body
9	Vitreous chamber
10	Fundus
11	Sclera
12	M. retractor bulbi
13	Mm. recti
14	Optic nerve
15	Periorbita
16	M. temporalis

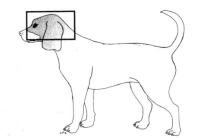

54

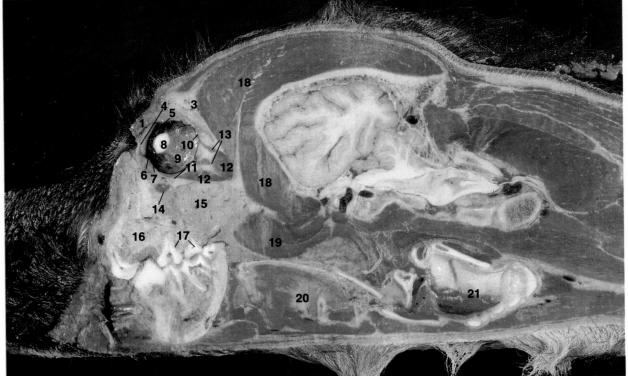

54 Lateral aspect of a sagittal section through the head of a dog. The structure of the eyeball and the orbital contents are shown.

1	Upper eyelid (palpebra superior)
2	Medial commissure
3	Frontal bone
4	Conjunctival sac
5	Cornea
6	Anterior chamber
7	Ciliary body
8	Lens
9	Vitreous chamber
10	Retinal layer
11	Choroid
12	Mm. recti
13	M. retractor bulbi
14	M. obliquus ventralis
15	Zygomatic gland
16	Maxilla
17	Upper molar teeth
18	M. temporalis
19	M. pterygoideus
20	Tongue
21	Larynx

• This section of the head gives an anatomical plane similar to that in a vertical ultrasound scan of the eye.

55

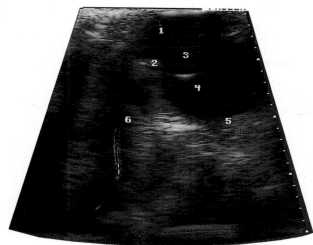

55 Ultrasound scan of the eye of a dog, demonstrating the contents of the bulb of the eye (eyeball). The plane of the scan is vertical and corresponds to **54**. The caudal surface of the lens is indicated by a white line between 3 and 4, which is due to specular reflection from the lens surface.

1	Anterior chamber	4	Vitreous chamber
2	Ciliary body	5	Optic disc region
3	Lens	6	Ventral aspect of orbit

56

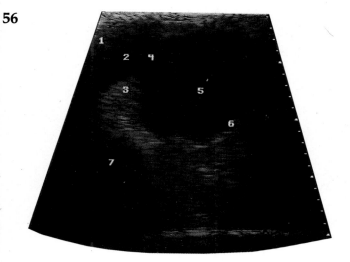

56 Ultrasound scan of the eye of a dog, demonstrating the contents of the bulb of the eye. The healthy lens is almost echolucent, but its position is marked (4). The plane of the scan is horizontal and corresponds to **53**.

1	Corneal surface	6	Caudal scleral surface
2	Anterior chamber		(with retrobulbar
3	Ciliary body		contents distal to it)
4	Lens	7	Medial aspect of orbit
5	Vitreous chamber		

57

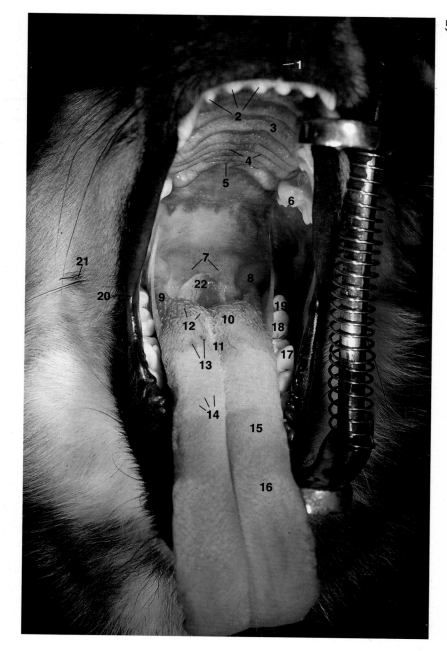

57 Rostral aspect of the open oral cavity, revealing the structures of the caudal oral cavity.

1	Philtrum	12	Filiform papillae
2	Upper incisor teeth	13	Vallate papillae
3	Hard palate	14	Fungiform papillae
4	Palatine ridges	15	Body ⎫ of tongue
5	Palatine raphe	16	Dorsal face ⎭
6	Fourth upper premolar (carnassial) tooth	17	First ⎫
7	Soft palate	18	Second ⎬ lower molar tooth
8	Palatine tonsils in crypt	19	Third ⎭
9	Palatoglossal arch	20	Angle of mouth
10	Root of tongue	21	Vibrissae
11	Median groove	22	Epiglottis

- This is the view exposed prior to endotracheal intubation of the dog. The soft palate is then elevated to expose the aditus laryngis.

41

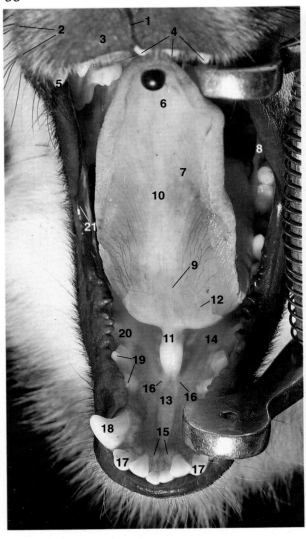

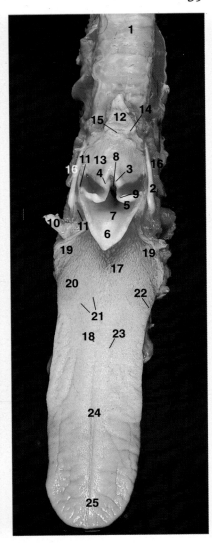

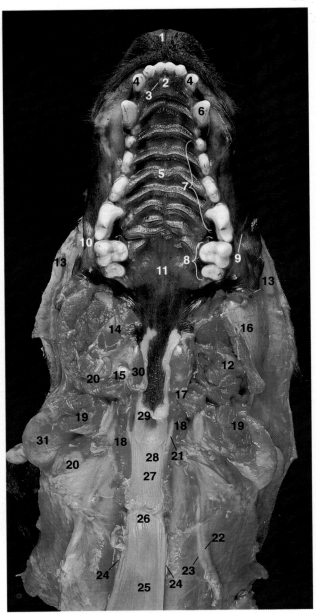

58 Rostral aspect of the oral cavity of a dog. The tongue has been elevated dorsally to reveal the ventral floor of the oral cavity.

1	Philtrum
2	Tactile hairs
3	Upper lip (labia superior)
4	Upper incisor teeth
5	Upper canine tooth
6	Apex } of tongue
7	Ventral face
8	Buccal vestibule
9	Lingual vein
10	Position of lyssa
11	Sublingual frenulum
12	Fimbriated plica
13	Sublingual recess
14	Lateral sublingual recess
15	Orobasal organ
16	Sublingual caruncle with opening of mandibular duct and major sublingual duct
17	Lower incisor teeth
18	Lower canine tooth
19	First and second lower premolar teeth
20	Gums
21	Angle of mouth

59 Dorsal aspect of the tongue and larynx of a dog.

1	Trachea
2	Dorsal border of thyroid cartilage
3	Corniculate process of arytenoid cartilage
4	Corniculate } tubercle
5	Cuneiform
6	Epiglottis
7	Laryngeal inlet
8	Interarytenoid groove
9	Aryepiglottic fold
10	Hyoid bone
11	Piriform recess
12	Oesophagus
13	Caudal part of laryngopharynx
14	Pharyngo-oesphageal junction
15	Limen pharyngoesophageum
16	Palatopharyngeal arch
17	Root } of tongue
18	Body
19	Palatopharyngeal arch
20	Filiform papillae
21	Vallate papillae
22	Foliate papillae
23	Fungiform papillae
24	Median groove (sulcus)
25	Apex of tongue

60 Ventral aspect of a section of the head of a dog, made in the dorsal plane through the digestive tube.

1	Philtrum	17	Hypoglossal nerve
2	Incisive papilla	18	Pharyngeal muscles
3	Orifice of incisive duct	19	M. digastricus
4	Incisor teeth	20	Mandibular lymph node
5	Hard palate	21	Thyroid cartilage
6	Canine teeth	22	Common carotid artery
7	Premolar teeth	23	Vagosympathetic trunk
8	Molar teeth	24	Thyroid gland
9	Orifice of parotid duct	25	Oesophagus
10	Region of orifices of zygomatic ducts	26	Annular fold
11	Soft palate	27	Dorsal wall of laryngeal pharynx
12	Mandible	28	Pharyngeal isthmus
13	M. buccinator	29	Pharyngopalatine arch
14	M. styloglossus	30	Palatine tonsil
15	Epihyoid bone	31	Mandibular salivary gland
16	M. masseter		

61 Lateral radiograph of the head of a dog. To demonstrate the position of the mandibular salivary gland, radio-opaque material has been injected into the duct of the gland.

1 Needle inserted into orifice of duct of mandibular salivary gland at sublingual caruncle
2 Duct of mandibular salivary gland
3 Mandibular salivary gland
4 Hyoid bone

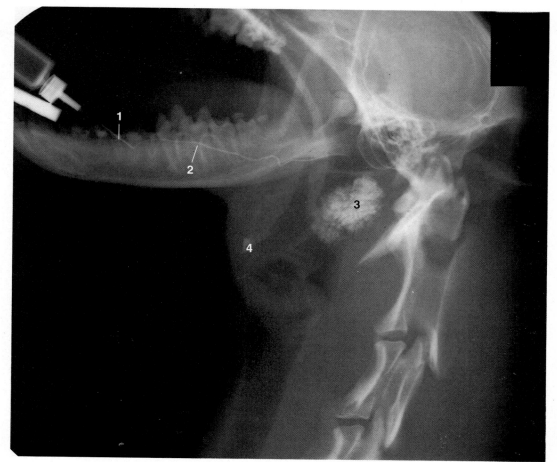

62 Lateral radiograph of the head of a dog. Radio-opaque material has been injected into the duct of the monostomatic sublingual salivary gland to outline its course and the glandular tissue.

1 Needle inserted into orifice of duct of monostomatic sublingual salivary gland at sublingual caruncle
2 Duct of monostomatic sublingual salivary gland
3 Glandular tissue around duct
4 Portion of monostomatic sublingual salivary gland encapsulated with mandibular salivary gland
5 Endotracheal tube
6 Hyoid bone

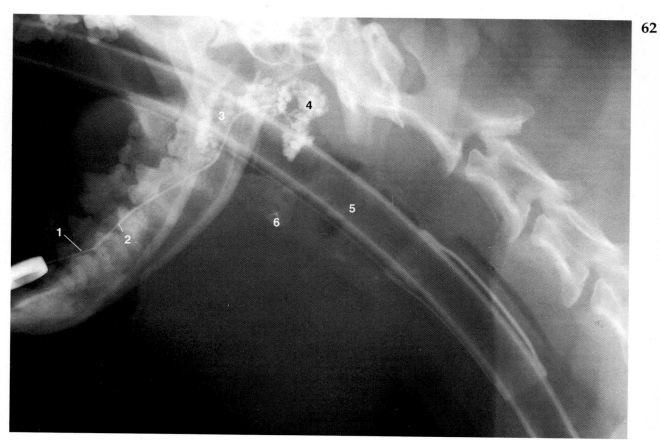

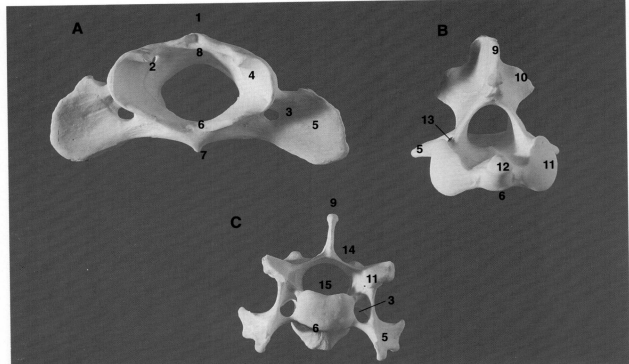

63 Cranial aspect of the first (atlas) (A), second (axis) (B), and fifth cervical vertebrae (C) of a dog.

1	Dorsal tubercle
2	Lateral vertebral foramen
3	Transverse foramen
4	Cranial articular fovea
5	Transverse process (wing of atlas)
6	Body
7	Ventral tubercle
8	Dorsal arch
9	Spinous process
10	Caudal articular process
11	Cranial articular surface
12	Dens (odontoid process)
13	Transverse canal
14	Lamina
15	Vertebral foramen

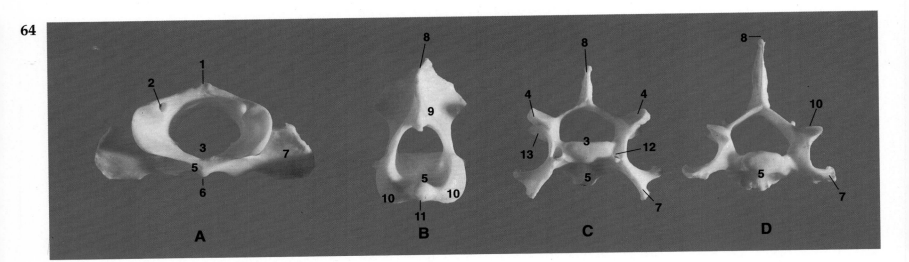

64 Cranial aspect of the first (atlas) (A), second (axis) (B), fifth (C) and seventh cervical vertebrae (D) of a cat.

1	Dorsal tubercle	6	Ventral tubercle	11	Dens (odontoid process)
2	Lateral vertebral foramen	7	Transverse process (wing of atlas)	12	Transverse foramen
3	Vertebral foramen	8	Spinous process	13	Caudal articular process
4	Cranial articular fovea	9	Arch		
5	Body	10	Cranial articular surface		

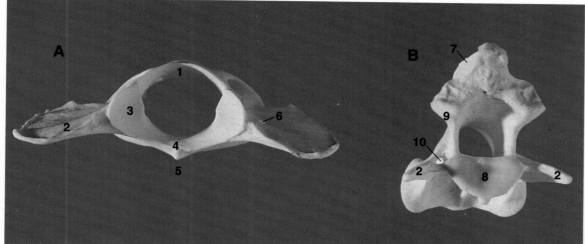

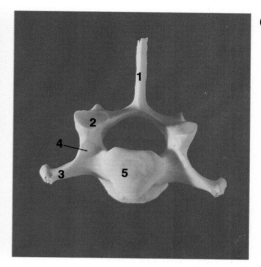

65 Caudal aspect of the first (atlas) (A) and second (axis) (B) cervical vertebrae of a dog.

1	Arch	6	Transverse foramen
2	Transverse process	7	Spinous process
3	Caudal articular fovea	8	Body of axis
4	Fovea for dens (odontoid process)	9	Caudal articular process
5	Ventral tubercle	10	Transverse foramen

66 Cranial aspect of the seventh cervical vertebra of a dog.

1	Spinous process
2	Cranial articular surface
3	Transverse process
4	Transverse foramen
5	Body

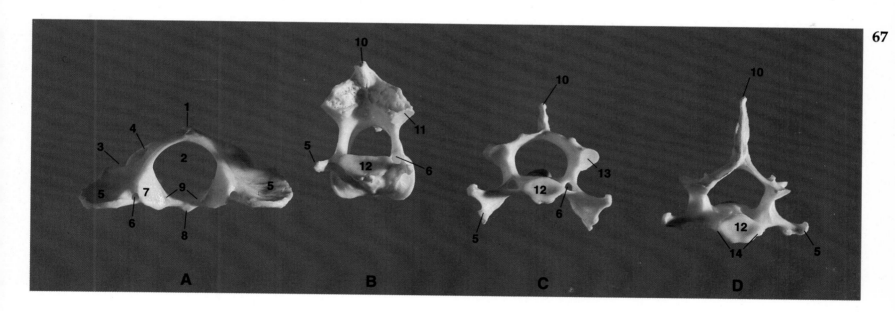

67 Caudal aspect of the first (atlas) (A), second (axis) (B), fifth (C) and seventh cervical vertebrae (D) of a cat.

1	Dorsal tubercle	6	Transverse foramen	11	Caudal articular surface
2	Vertebral foramen	7	Caudal articular fovea	12	Body
3	Alar notch	8	Ventral tubercle	13	Caudal articular surface
4	Lateral vertebral foramen	9	Fovea of dens	14	Caudal costal fovea
5	Transverse process	10	Spinous process		

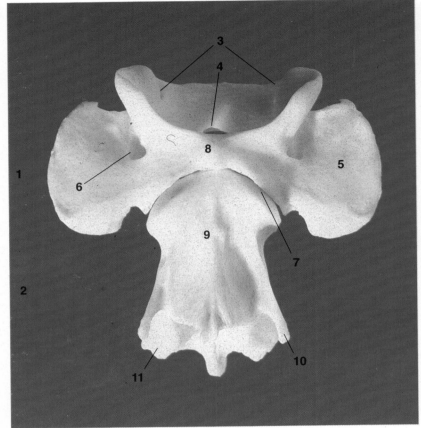

68 Ventral aspect of the first (atlas) and second (axis) cervical vertebrae of a cat.

69 Dorsal aspect of the first (A) (atlas), second (axis) (B), and third (C) cervical vertebrae of a cat.

1	Atlas	7	Atlantoaxial articulation
2	Axis	8	Ventral tubercle
3	Cranial articular fovea	9	Body
4	Dens (odontoid process)	10	Transverse process
5	Wing of atlas	11	Caudal articular surface
6	Transverse foramen		

1	Lateral vertebral foramen	4	Spinous process
2	Alar notch	5	Atlantoaxial articulation
3	Transverse process	6	Caudal articular process

70 Lateral aspect of the first cervical vertebra (atlas) of a dog.

1	Dorsal tubercle	4	Transverse process (wing of atlas)
2	Arch	5	Transverse foramen
3	Lateral vertebral foramen	6	Ventral tubercle

71 Lateral aspect of the second cervical vertebra (axis) of a dog.

1 Spinous process	6 Transverse foramen
2 Arch	7 Caudal articular process
3 Dens (odontoid process)	8 Transverse process
4 Cranial articular surface	9 Median ventral crest
5 Body	

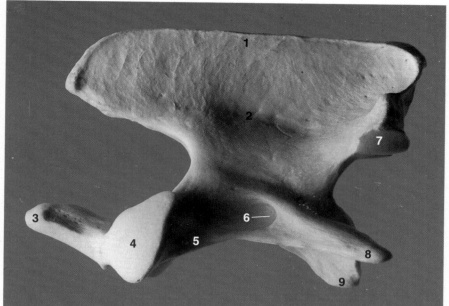

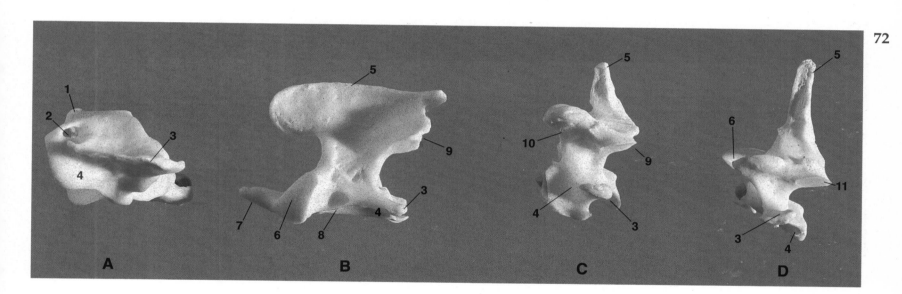

72 Left lateral aspect of the first (atlas) (A), second (axis) (B), fifth (C) and seventh (D) cervical vertebrae of a cat.

1 Dorsal tubercle	5 Spinous process	9 Caudal articular process
2 Lateral vertebral foramen	6 Cranial articular surface	10 Cranial articular process
3 Transverse process	7 Dens (odontoid process)	11 Caudal articular surface
4 Body	8 Transverse foramen	

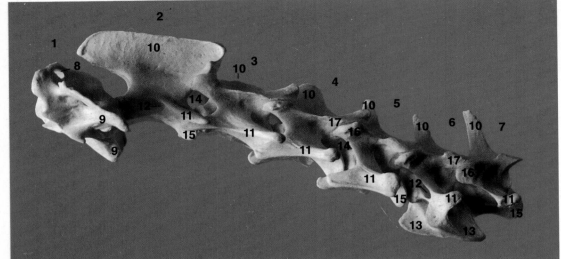

73 Lateral aspect of the articulated cervical vertebrae of a dog.

1	First (atlas)	cervical vertebrae
2	Second (axis)	
3	Third	
4	Fourth	
5	Fifth	
6	Sixth	
7	Seventh	
8	Lateral vertebral foramen	
9	Wing of 1	
10	Spinous process	
11	Transverse process	
12	Transverse foramen	
13	Expanded plate of transverse process of 6	
14	Intervertebral foramen	
15	Body	
16	Cranial articular process	
17	Caudal articular process	

74

74 Dorsal aspect of the articulated cervical vertebrae of a dog.

1	First (atlas)	cervical vertebrae
2	Second (axis)	
3	Third	
4	Fourth	
5	Fifth	
6	Sixth	
7	Seventh	
8	Arch	
9	Lateral vertebral foramen	
10	Alar notch	
11	Wing of 1	
12	Transverse foramen	
13	Spinous process	
14	Transverse process	
15	Expanded plate of transverse process of 6	
16	Cranial articular process	
17	Caudal articular process	
18	Body	
19	Dens	
20	Atlantoaxial articulation	

75

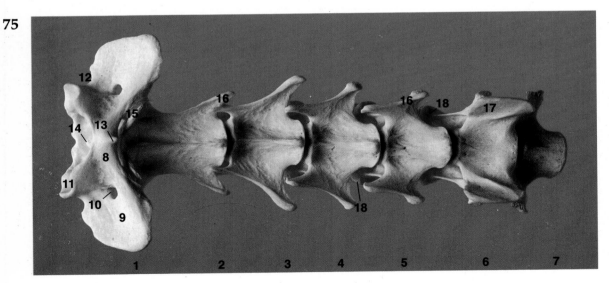

75 Ventral aspect of the articulated cervical vertebrae of a dog.

1	First (atlas)	cervical vertebrae
2	Second (axis)	
3	Third	
4	Fourth	
5	Fifth	
6	Sixth	
7	Seventh	
8	Body	
9	Wing	
10	Transverse foramen	
11	Cranial articular fovea	
12	Alar notch	
13	Ventral tubercle	
14	Dens	
15	Atlantoaxial articulation	
16	Transverse process	
17	Expanded plate of transverse process of 6	
18	Cranial articular process	

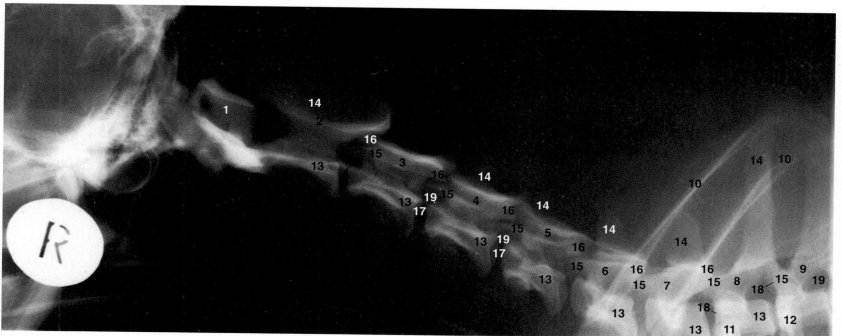

76 Lateral radiograph of the cervical portion of the vertebral column of a dog.

1	First (atlas)	
2	Second (axis)	
3	Third	
4	Fourth	cervical
5	Fifth	vertebrae
6	Sixth	
7	Seventh	
8	First	} thoracic vertebrae
9	Second	
10	Scapula	
11	First	} rib
12	Second	
13	Body	
14	Spinous process	
15	Cranial articular process	
16	Caudal articular process	
17	Location of intervertebral disc	
18	Fovea for articulation of rib	
19	Intervertebral foramen	

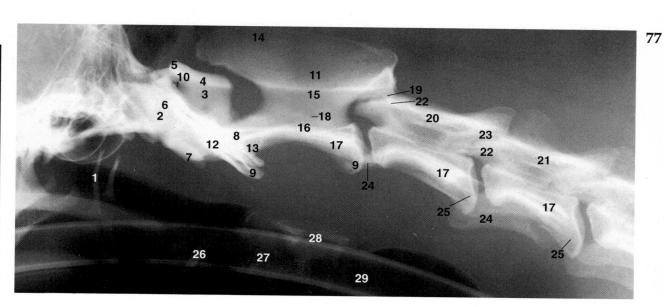

77 Lateral radiograph of the cranial cervical portion of the vertebral column of a dog.

1	Stylohyoid bone	15	Dorsal border } of vertebral foramen
2	Occipital condyle	16	Ventral border } (vertebral canal)
3	First cervical vertebra (atlas)	17	Body
4	Dorsal arch	18	Transverse foramen
5	Dorsal tubercle	19	Articular processes
6	Border of cranial articular surface	20	Third } cervical vertebra
7	Ventral arch	21	Fourth
8	Border of caudal articular surface	22	Cranial articular process
9	Transverse process	23	Caudal articular process
10	Lateral vertebral foramen	24	Cranial extension } of transverse process
11	Second cervical vertebra (axis)	25	Caudal extension
12	Dens	26	Thyrohyoid bone
13	Cranial articular surface	27	Thyroid cartilage
14	Spinous process	28	Cricoid cartilage
		29	Trachea (with endotracheal tube)

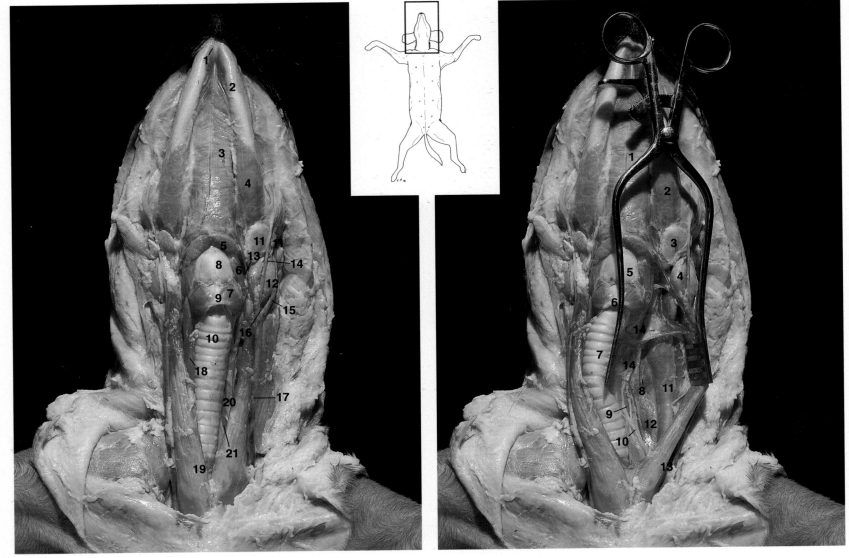

78 Ventral aspect of the deep structures of the neck of a dog. The ventral muscles have been resected to expose the trachea.

79 Ventral aspect of the deep structures of the neck of a dog. The trachea has been deviated from the midline to reveal the oesophagus and carotid sheath.

1	Mandibular symphysis	13	Lingual vein
2	Mandibular body	14	Facial vein
3	M. mylohyoideus	15	Maxillary vein
4	M. digastricus	16	Linguofacial vein
5	M. sternohyoideus (cut edge)	17	External jugular vein
6	M. thyrohyoideus	18	M. sternothyroideus
7	M. cricothyroideus	19	M. sternocephalicus
8	Thyroid cartilage	20	Carotid sheath with vagosympathetic trunk, carotid artery and internal jugular vein
9	Cricoid cartilage		
10	Tracheal rings		
11	Mandibular lymph nodes	21	Recurrent laryngeal nerve
12	Mandibular salivary gland		

1	M. mylohyoideus	8	Carotid artery
2	M. digastricus	9	Vagosympathetic trunk
3	Mandibular lymph node	10	Recurrent laryngeal nerve
4	Mandibular salivary gland	11	Oesophagus
5	Thyroid cartilage	12	M. longus colli
6	Cricoid cartilage	13	M. sternocephalicus
7	Trachea diverted to right	14	Thyroid gland

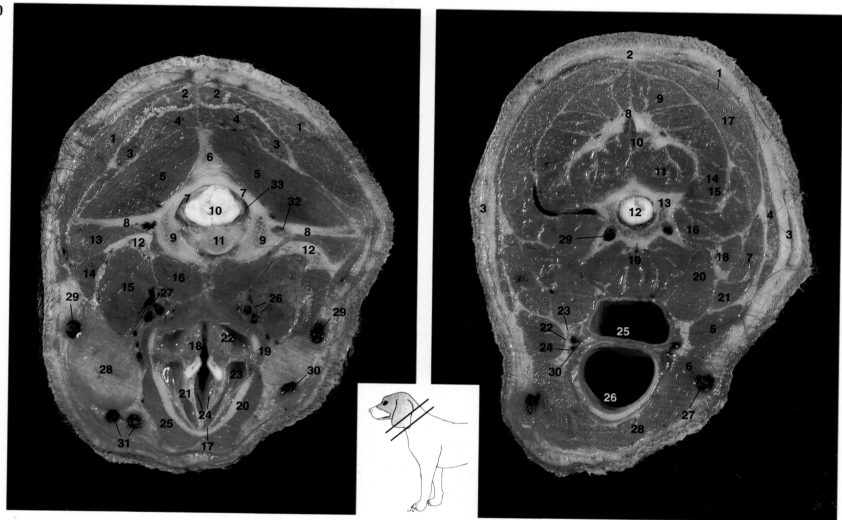

80 Cranial aspect of a transverse section through the neck of a dog at the level of the atlantoaxial joint.

81 Cranial aspect of a transverse section through the neck of a dog at the level of the third cervical vertebra.

1	M. splenius capitis
2	M. semispinalis capitis (biventer)
3	M. semispinalis capitis (complexus)
4	M. rectus capitis dorsalis major
5	M. obliquus capitis caudalis
6	Spinous process of second cervical vertebra (axis)
7	Arch ⎤ of first cervical
8	Wing ⎬ vertebra (atlas)
9	Body ⎦
10	Spinal cord
11	Dens (odontoid process) of second cervical vertebra (axis)
12	Jugular process
13	Mm. intertransversarii cervicis
14	M. omotransversarius
15	M. longus capitis
16	M. rectus capitis ventralis
17	Larynx
18	Arytenoid cartilages
19	Cricoid cartilage
20	Thyroid cartilage
21	Vocal folds
22	M. cricoarytenoideus dorsalis
23	Lateral ventricle
24	Rima glottis
25	M. thyrohyoideus
26	Division of common carotid artery into external and internal carotid arteries
27	Vagosympathetic trunk
28	Mandibular salivary gland
29	Maxillary vein
30	Linguofacial vein
31	Linguofacial and facial veins (divided)
32	Vertebral artery and vein
33	Internal vertebral plexus

1	M. rhomboideus capitis
2	Dorsal median raphe
3	Mm. cutanei colli
4	M. brachiocephalicus (M. cleidocephalicus, pars cervicalis)
5	M. sternocephalicus, pars occipitalis, and M. cleidocephalicus, pars mastoidea
6	M. sternocephalicus, pars mastoidea
7	M. omotransversarius
8	Ligamentum nuchae
9	M. semispinalis capitis (biventer and complexus)
10	M. multifidus cervicis
11	M. spinalis cervicis
12	Spinal cord
13	Third cervical vertebra
14	Mm. longissimus capitis and atlantis
15	M. longissimus cervicis
16	Mm. intertransversarius dorsalis, medius and ventralis
17	M. splenius
18	M. serratus ventralis cervicis
19	M. longus colli
20	M. longus capitis
21	M. scalenus medius
22	Common carotid artery
23	Vagosympathetic trunk
24	Internal jugular vein
25	Oesophagus
26	Trachea
27	External jugular vein
28	M. sternohyoideus and M. sternothyroideus
29	Vertebral artery and vein
30	Recurrent laryngeal nerve

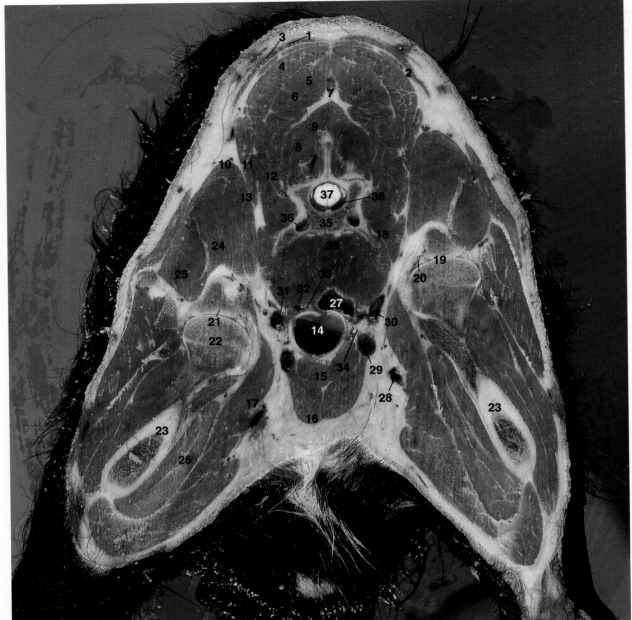

1	M. rhomboideus
2	Mm. cutanei colli
3	M. trapezius
4	M. splenius
5	M. biventer
6	M. complexus
7	Ligamentum nuchae
8	M. multifidus cervicis
9	M. spinalis cervicis
10	M. serratus ventralis cervicis
11	M. longissimus cervicis
12	Mm. longissimus capitis and atlantis
13	M. omotransversarius
14	Trachea
15	M. sternohyoideus and M. sternothyroideus
16	M. sternocephalicus
17	M. brachiocephalicus (M. cleidobrachialis)
18	Mm. intertransversarii
19	Shoulder joint
20	Joint capsule
21	Glenoid surface of scapula
22	Head } of humerus
23	Body
24	M. supraspinatus
25	M. infraspinatus
26	M. biceps brachii
27	Oesophagus
28	Cephalic vein
29	Jugular vein
30	Superficial cervical vein
31	Common carotid artery
32	Internal jugular vein
33	Vagosympathetic trunk
34	Recurrent laryngeal nerve
35	Seventh cervical vertebra
36	Vertebral artery and vein
37	Spinal cord
38	Internal vertebral plexus
39	M. longus colli

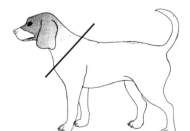

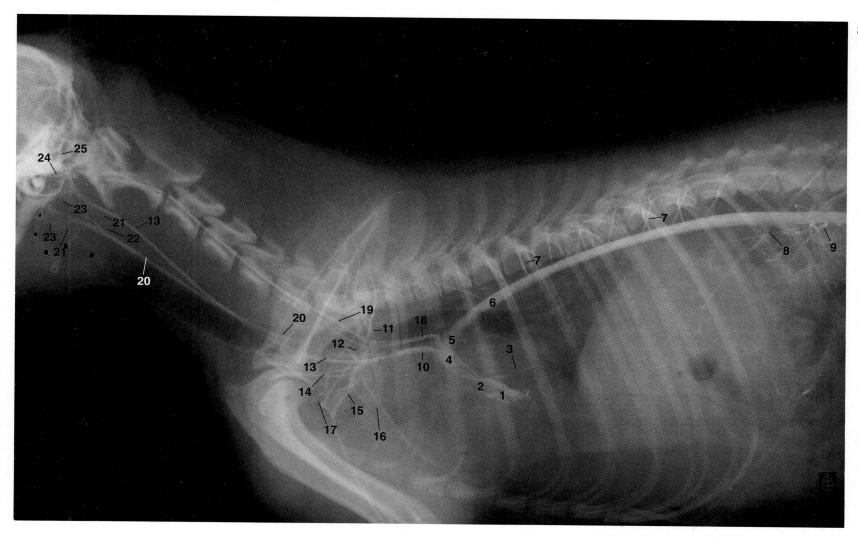

83 Lateral radiograph of an arteriogram of the major arterial vessels to the head and neck of a dog.

1	Left ventricular outflow tract	10	Brachiocephalic trunk	19	Left vertebral artery
2	Aortic valve	11	Right costocervical trunk	20	Left common carotid artery
3	Coronary artery	12	Right vertebral artery	21	Cranial laryngeal artery
4	Ascending aorta	13	Right common carotid artery	22	Internal carotid artery
5	Aortic arch	14	Right subclavian artery	23	Lingual artery
6	Descending aorta	15	Axillary artery	24	Facial artery
7	Segmental arteries	16	Internal thoracic artery	25	Maxillary artery
8	Coeliac artery	17	External thoracic artery		
9	Cranial mesenteric artery	18	Left subclavian artery		

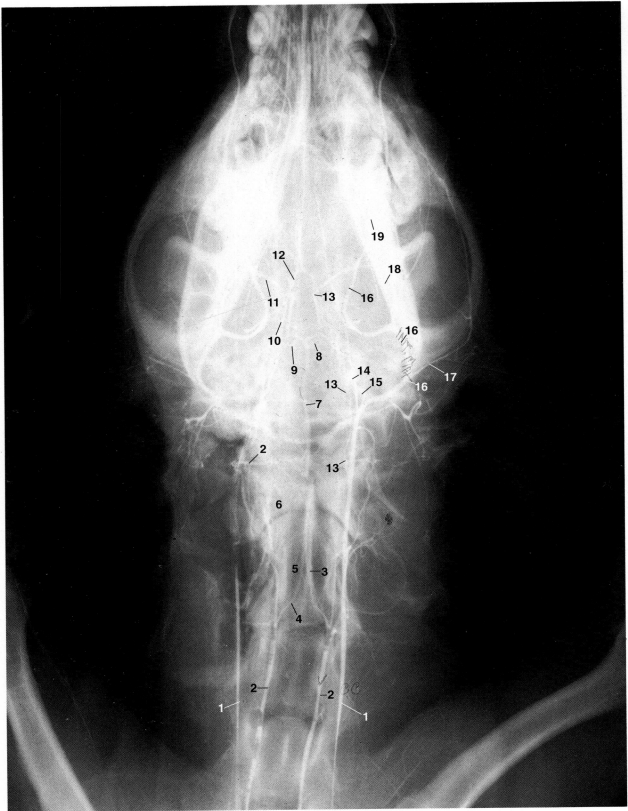

1	Common carotid artery
2	Vertebral artery
3	Ventral spinal artery
4	Spinal ramus
5	Second cervical vertebra (axis)
6	First cervical vertebra (atlas)
7	Basilar artery
8	Caudal communicating artery
9	Rostral cerebellar artery
10	Caudal cerebral artery
11	Middle cerebral artery
12	Rostral cerebral artery
13	Internal carotid artery
14	Lingual artery
15	Facial artery
16	Maxillary artery
17	Superficial temporal artery
18	Mandibular alveolar artery
19	Infra orbital artery

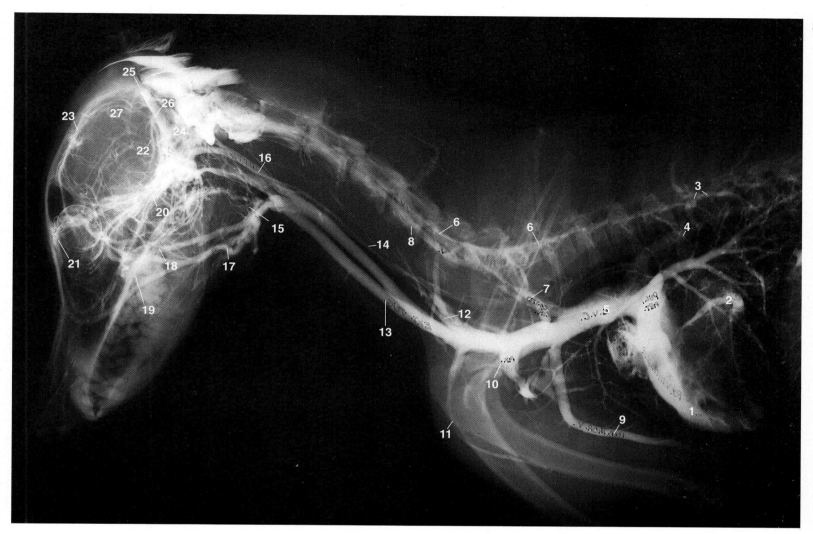

85 Lateral radiograph of a venogram of the head and neck of a dog.

1	Right ventricle	15	Linguofacial vein
2	Coronary veins	16	Maxillary vein
3	Intercostal veins	17	Lingual vein
4	Azygos vein	18	Deep facial vein
5	Cranial vena cava	19	Facial vein
6	Internal vertebral venous plexus	20	Cavernous sinus
7	Costocervical vein	21	Angular vein of eye
8	Vertebral vein	22	Temporal sinus
9	Internal thoracic vein	23	Dorsal sagittal sinus
10	Axillary vein	24	Straight sinus
11	Cephalic vein	25	Transverse sinus
12	Superficial cervical vein	26	Sigmoid sinus
13	External jugular vein	27	Dorsal petrosal sinus
14	Internal jugular vein		

3 Spinal column

Using bony specimens and radiographs, the osteology of the vertebral column is demonstrated in the other chapters of the book, where such detail is more relevant to the understanding of the anatomy of the respective regions. This short chapter is designed to illustrate the particular musculature surrounding the spinal column, together with the contents of the vertebral canal, by means of fresh dissected material.

86 Lateral aspect of the superficial epaxial muscles and the muscles of the thoracic cage of a dog. The left thoracic limb with its extrinsic muscles has been removed, as has the cutaneous trunci muscle.

1	M. splenius cervicis
2	M. longissimus cervicis
3	M. serratus dorsalis cranialis
4	M. longissimus thoracis
5	M. spinalis and semispinalis
6	Mm. longissimus thoracis and lumborum
7	M. iliocostalis
8	Mm. intercostales
9	M. scalenus
10	Trachea
11	M. sternothyroideus
12	M. sternocephalicus
13	External jugular vein
14	Mm. pectorales superficiales (cut)
15	M. pectoralis profundus (cut)
16	M. rectus abdominis
17	M. obliquus externus abdominis
18	Distal lateral cutaneous branches of intercostal nerves
19	Manubrium sterni
20	Costochondral joints
21	Sternocostal joints

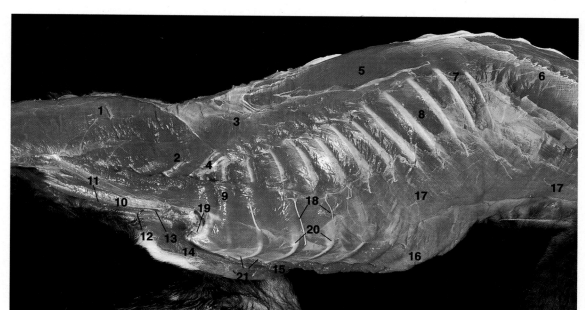

87 Lateral aspect of the deep epaxial muscles of the trunk of a dog. The dorsal serratus cranialis muscle has been removed.

1	Lumbodorsal fascia (cut)
2	Mm. longissimus thoracis and lumborum
3	M. obliquus externus abdominis
4	M. obliquus internus abdominis
5	M. rectus abdominis
6	M. iliocostalis lumborum
7	M. iliocostalis thoracis
8	M. longissimus cervicis
9	M. spinalis capitis
10	M. semispinalis capitis
11	M. spinalis and M. semispinalis thoracis

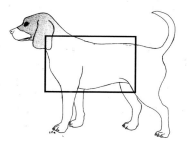

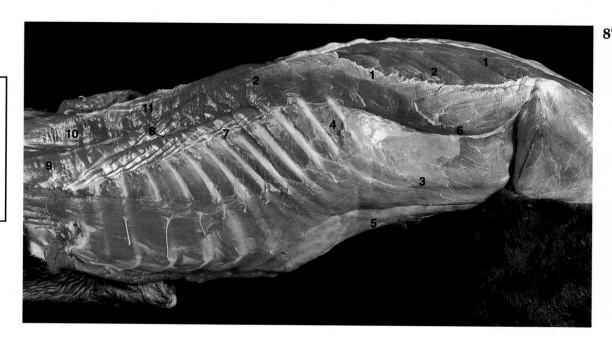

88

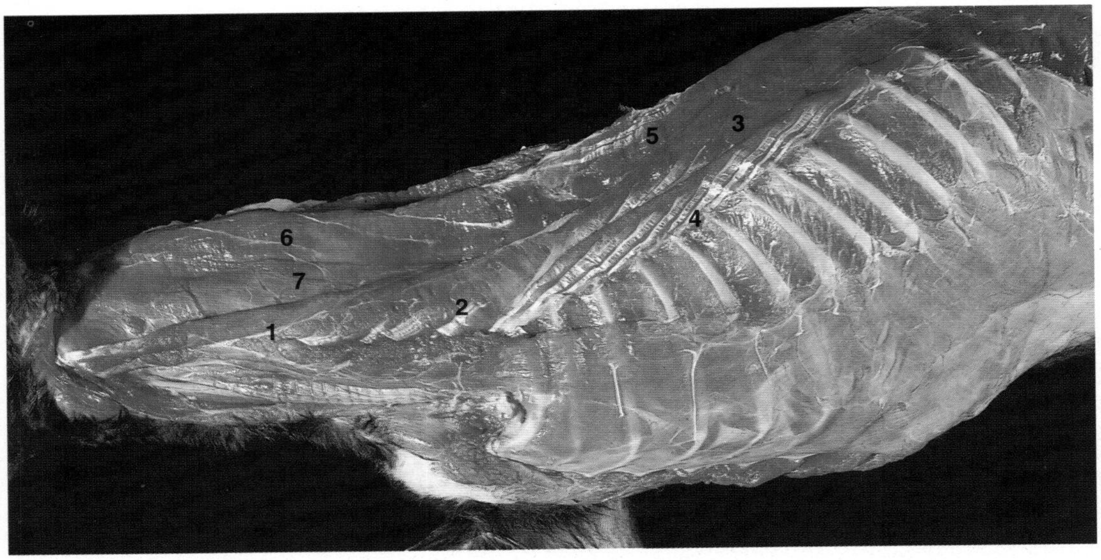

88 Lateral aspect of the deep epaxial muscles of the neck and thoracic region of a dog. The splenius cervicis and dorsal serratus cranialis muscles have been removed.

1 M. longissimus capitis
2 M. longissimus cervicis
3 Mm. longissimus thoracis and lumborum
4 M. iliocostalis thoracis
5 M. spinalis and M. semispinalis thoracis
6 M. semispinalis capitis (biventer)
7 M. semispinalis capitis (complexus)

89

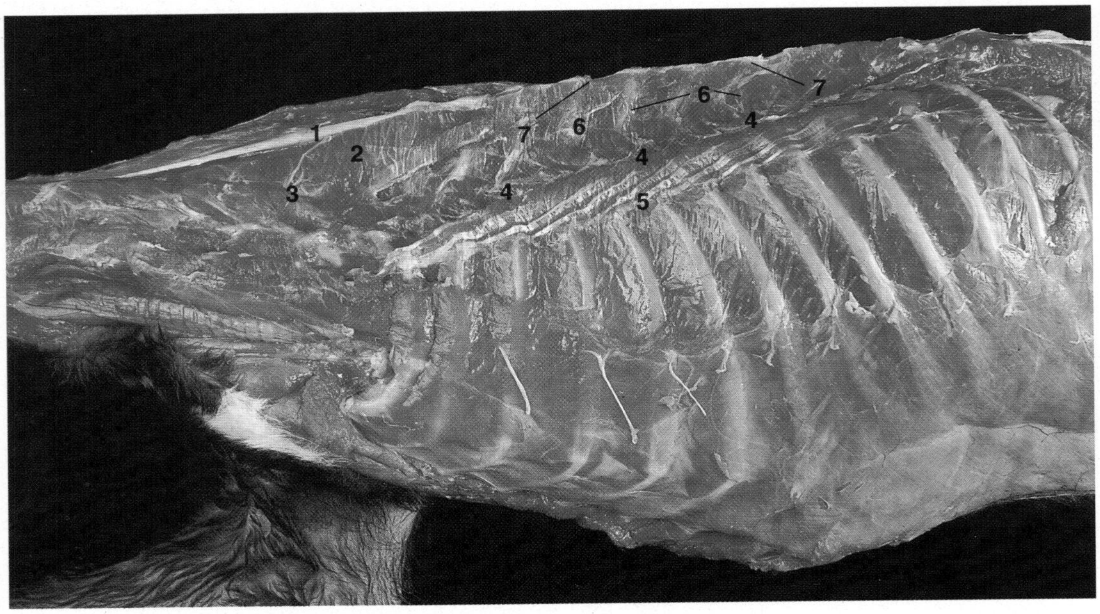

89 Lateral aspect of the deeper layer of the epaxial muscles of the neck and thorax of a dog. The semispinalis capitis and thoracis muscles have been removed to expose the ligamentum nuchae.

1 Ligamentum nuchae
2 M. spinalis cervicis
3 M. multifidus cervicis
4 M. multifidus thoracis
5 M. iliocostalis thoracis
6 Mm. interspinales
7 Supraspinous ligament

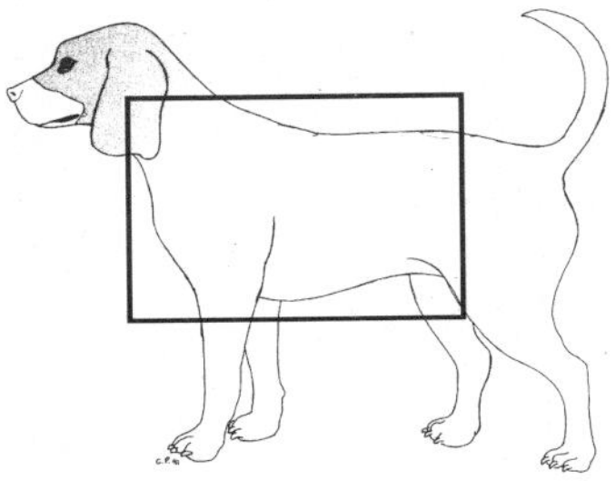

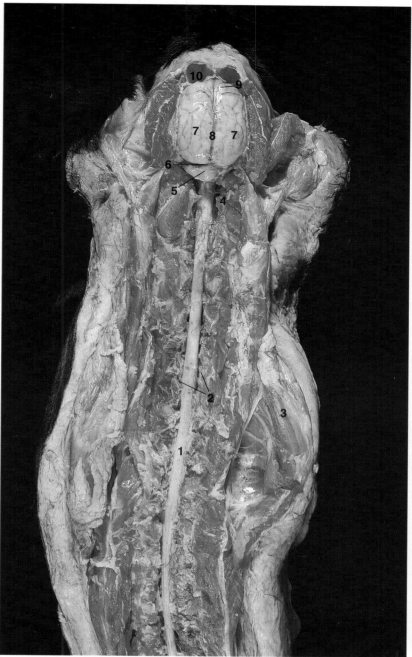

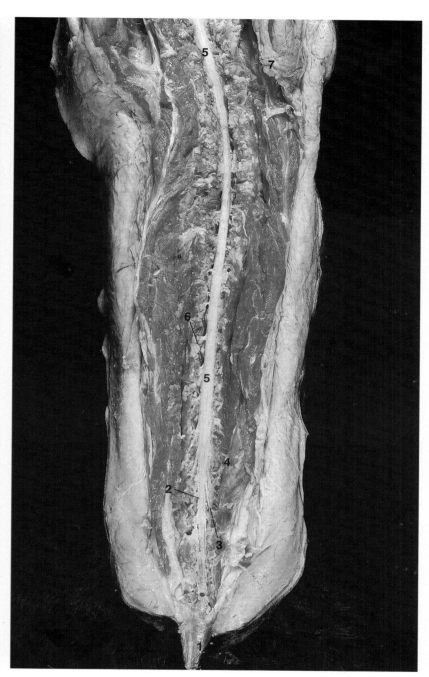

90 Dorsal aspect of the brain and spinal cord of a dog, to the level of the thoracolumbar junction. The dorsal epaxial muscles, the dorsal vertebral laminae, and the root of the cranium have been removed to reveal the meningeal layers covering the brain and spinal cord.

1	Dura mater covering spinal cord		transverse fissure
2	Vertebral canal	7	Cerebral hemispheres
3	Pectoral limb	8	Sagittal sinus overlying
4	First cervical vertebra (atlas)		longitudinal fissure
5	Cerebellum	9	Olfactory bulbs
6	Transverse sinus overlying	10	Frontal sinus

91 Dorsal aspect of the spinal cord of a dog, from the level of the first thoracic vertebra. The dorsal epaxial muscles and the dorsal vertebral laminae have been removed to reveal the vertebral canal.

1	Tail	5	Dura mater covering spinal cord
2	Cauda equina	6	Spinal nerve
3	Caudal spinal nerves	7	Pectoral limb
4	Sacrum		

4 Thoracic limb

Beginning with the proximal structures and descending distally to the manus, the osteology and myology of the thoracic limb are displayed. The osteological details are revealed first, using bony specimens (both singly and in an articulated form) and radiographs, and the muscular attachments are then illustrated, followed by prepared dissections. Blood vessels and nerves are named as they occur in the dissections, and a contrast medium is used with radiography to explain the course of the vascular supply.

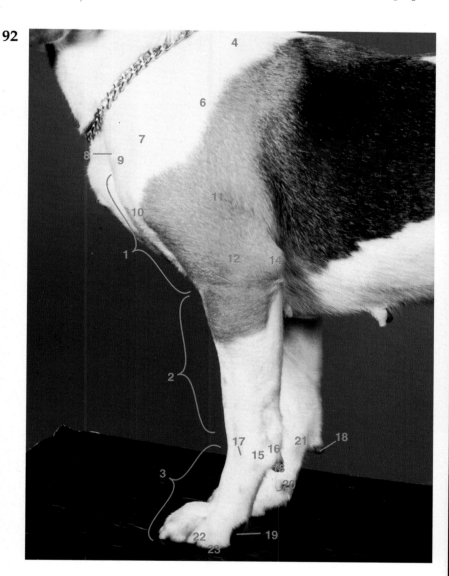

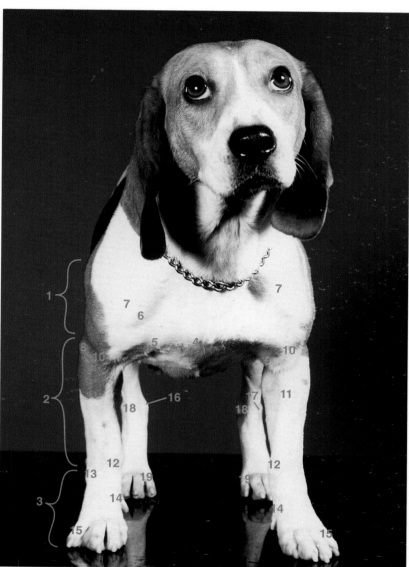

92 Lateral aspect of the left thoracic limb of a standing live dog, demonstrating palpable landmarks commonly used in clinical examination.

1	Brachium	13	Elbow joint (cubital joint)
2	Antebrachium	14	Olecranon process } of ulna
3	Manus	15	Styloid process } of ulna
4	Cranial angle } of scapula	16	Accessory carpal bone
5	Caudal angle } of scapula	17	Carpal joint
6	Spine	18	Carpal pad
7	Acromion	19	Metacarpal pad
8	Shoulder joint	20	First digit (dew claw)
9	Greater tubercle of humerus	21	Styloid process of radius
10	Deltoid tuberosity	22	Fifth digit
11	M. triceps brachii	23	Digital pad
12	Lateral epicondyle of humerus		

93 Cranial aspect of the thoracic limbs of a standing live dog, demonstrating palpable landmarks. The dorsal aspect of the pes of the pelvic limb is also displayed.

1	Brachium	11	Cephalic vein (in subcutaneous position)
2	Antebrachium	12	Styloid process of radius
3	Manus	13	Styloid process of ulna
4	Manubrium of sterni	14	First digit
5	Pectoral muscle mass	15	Fifth digit
6	M. brachiocephalicus	16	Medial malleolus of tibia
7	Shoulder joint	17	Lateral malleolus of fibula } pelvic
8	Lateral epicondyle } of humerus	18	Tarsal joint (hock) } limb
9	Medial epicondyle } of humerus	19	Second digit
10	Elbow joint		

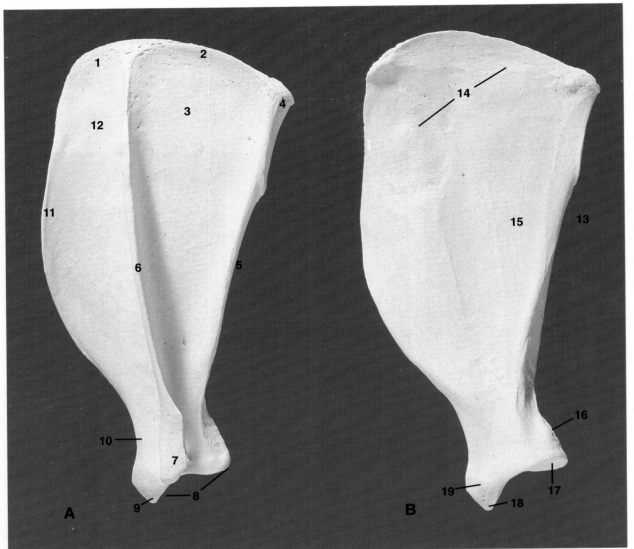

94 Lateral aspect of the left scapula (A) and medial aspect of the right scapula (B) of a dog.

1	Cranial angle
2	Dorsal border
3	Infraspinous fossa
4	Caudal angle
5	Caudal border
6	Spine
7	Acromion
8	Ventral angle
9	Supraglenoid tubercle
10	Scapular notch
11	Cranial border
12	Supraspinous fossa
13	Caudal border
14	Facies serrata
15	Subscapular fossa
16	Infraglenoid tubercle
17	Glenoid cavity
18	Supraglenoid tubercle
19	Coracoid process

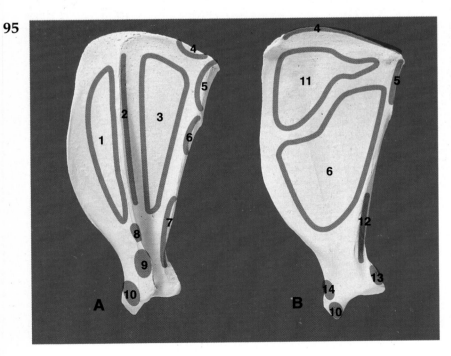

95 Lateral (A) and medial (B) aspect of the scapula of a dog, showing areas of muscle attachment.

1	Supraspinatus	8	Omotransversarius
2	Trapezius and deltoideus	9	Deltoideus
3	Infraspinatus	10	Biceps brachii
4	Rhomboideus	11	Serratus ventralis
5	Teres major	12	Long head of triceps
6	Subscapularis	13	Teres minor
7	Teres minor and long head of triceps	14	Coracobrachialis

96 Lateral (A) and medial (B) aspect of the scapula of a dog, showing the centres of ossification.

1	Body
2	Supraglenoid tubercle

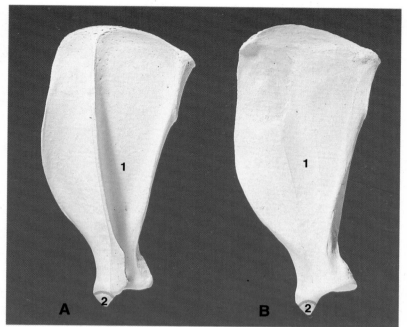

97 Lateral aspect of the left scapula (A) and medial aspect of the right scapula (B) of a cat.

1	Cranial angle
2	Dorsal border
3	Caudal angle
4	Infraspinous fossa
5	Caudal border
6	Spine
7	Tuberosity of spine
8	Suprahamate process ⎫ of acromion
9	Hamate process ⎭
10	Ventral angle
11	Supraglenoid tubercle
12	Scapular notch
13	Cranial border
14	Supraspinous fossa
15	Facies serrata
16	Subscapular fossa
17	Glenoid cavity
18	Coracoid process

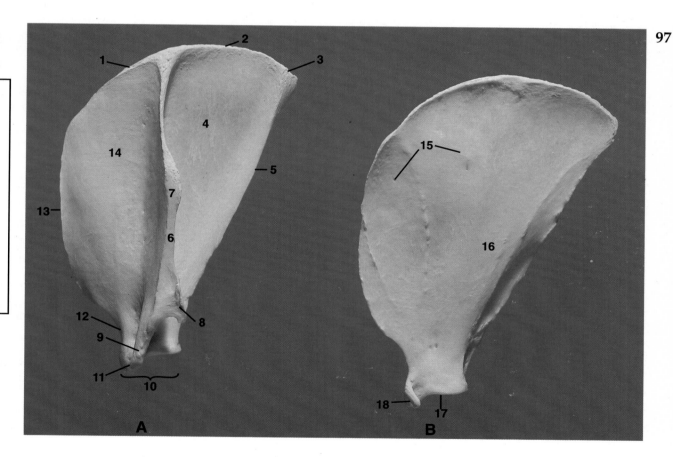

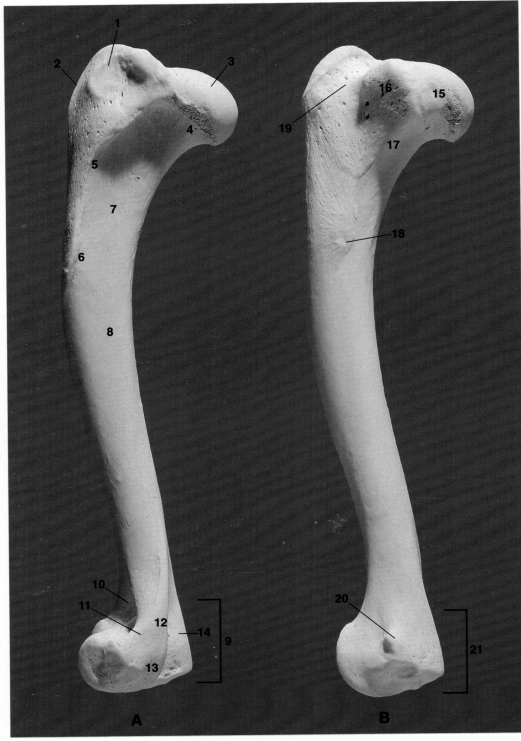

99 Lateral (A) and medial (B) aspect, of the humerus of a dog, showing areas of muscle attachment.

1	Supraspinatus
2	Infraspinatus
3	Teres minor
4	Accessory head of triceps
5	Brachialis
6	Lateral head of triceps
7	Deltoideus
8	Pectoralis superficialis
9	Cleidobrachialis
10	Brachioradialis
11	Extensor carpi radialis
12	Anconeus
13	Extensors of carpus and digits, and ulnaris lateralis
14	Supinator
15	Supraspinatus
16	Pectoralis profundus
17	Subscapularis
18	Coracobrachialis and medial head of triceps
19	Pronator teres
20	Flexors of carpus and digits
21	Teres major and latissimus dorsi

98 Lateral aspect of the left humerus (A) and medial aspect of the right humerus (B) of a dog.

1	Greater tubercle		(musculospiral groove)
2	Crest of 1	8	Body
3	Head	9	Condyle
4	Neck	10	Radial fossa
5	Tricipital line (anconeal crest)	11	Supratrochlear foramen
		12	Lateral epicondylar crest
6	Deltoid tuberosity	13	Lateral epicondyle
7	Brachial groove	14	Olecranon fossa

15	Head
16	Lesser tubercle
17	Crest of 16
18	Tuberosity for teres major
19	Intertubercular groove
20	Medial epicondyle
21	Condyle

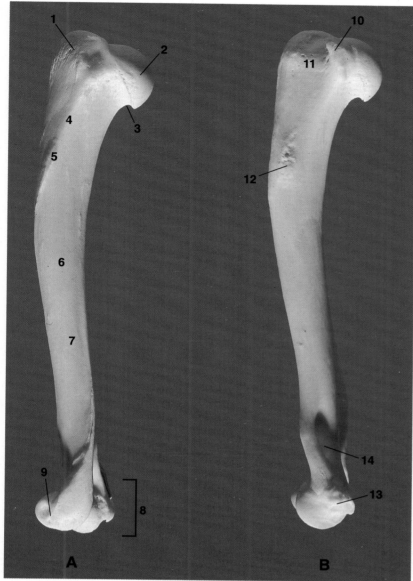

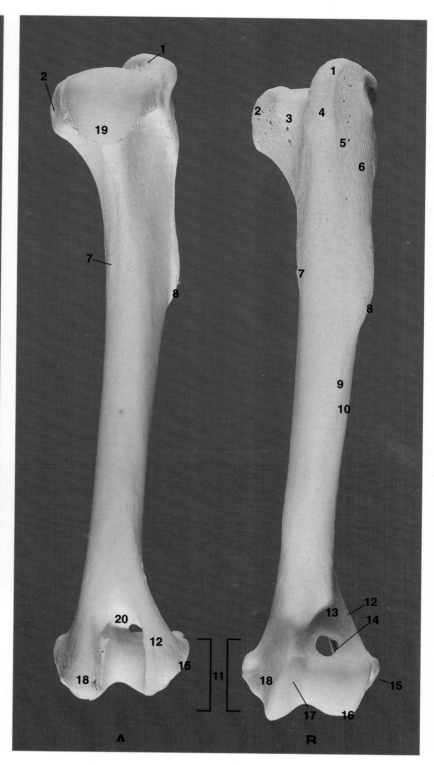

100 Lateral aspect of the left humerus (A) and medial aspect of the right humerus (B) of a cat.

1	Greater tubercle	8	Condyle
2	Head	9	Lateral epicondyle
3	Neck	10	Lesser tubercle
4	Tricipital line	11	Intertubercular groove
5	Deltoid tuberosity	12	Tuberosity for M. teres major
6	Body	13	Medial epicondyle
7	Brachial groove	14	Supracondylar foramen

101 Caudal aspect of the right humerus (A) and cranial aspect of the left humerus (B) of a dog.

1	Greater tubercle	8	Deltoid tuberosity	15	Lateral epicondyle
2	Lesser tubercle	9	Body	16	Capitulum
3	Intertubercular groove	10	Brachial groove	17	Trochlea
4	Crest of greater tubercle	11	Condyle	18	Medial epicondyle
5	Tuberosity for M. teres minor	12	Lateral epicondylar crest	19	Head
6	Tricipital line	13	Radial fossa	20	Olecranon fossa
7	Tuberosity for M. teres major	14	Supratrochlear foramen		

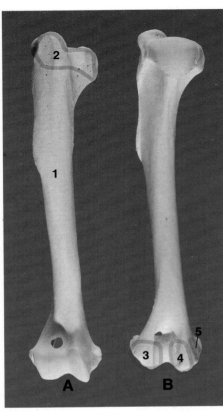

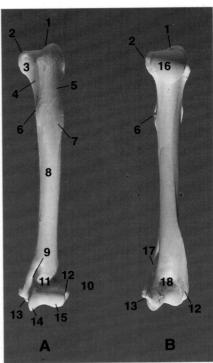

102 Cranial aspect of the right humerus (A) and caudal aspect of the lrft humerus (B) of a dog, showing the centres of ossification.

1	Body
2	Proximal
3	Lateral condyle
4	Medial condyle
5	Medial epicondyle

103 Cranial aspect of the left humerus (A) and caudal aspect of the right humerus (B) of a cat.

1	Greater tubercle
2	Lesser tubercle
3	Intertubercular groove
4	Crest of greater tubercle
5	Tricipital line
6	Tuberosity for M. teres major
7	Deltoid tuberosity
8	Body
9	Supracondylar foramen
10	Condyle
11	Radial fossa
12	Lateral epicondyle
13	Medial epicondyle
14	Trochlea
15	Capitulum
16	Head
17	Supracondylar foramen
18	Olecranon fossa

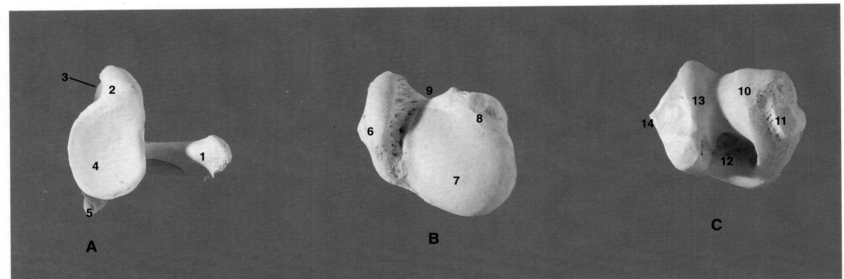

104 Distal extremity of the scapula (A), and proximal (B) and distal (C) extremities of the humerus of a dog.

1	Acromion process	6	Greater tubercle	11	Lateral epicondyle
2	Supraglenoid tubercle	7	Head	12	Olecranon fossa
3	Coracoid process	8	Lesser tubercle	13	Trochlea
4	Glenoid cavity	9	Intertubercular groove	14	Medial epicondyle
5	Infraglenoid tubercle	10	Capitulum		

**105 Cranial aspect of the left
shoulder joint (A) and caudal
aspect of the right shoulder joint
(B) of a dog.**

1	Body of scapula
2	Scapular spine
3	Acromion
4	Scapular notch
5	Supraglenoid tubercle
6	Coracoid process
7	Greater tubercle
8	Lesser tubercle
9	Intertubercular groove
10	Tricipital line
11	Body of humerus
12	Neck of scapula
13	Infraglenoid tubercle
14	Border of glenoid cavity
15	Head

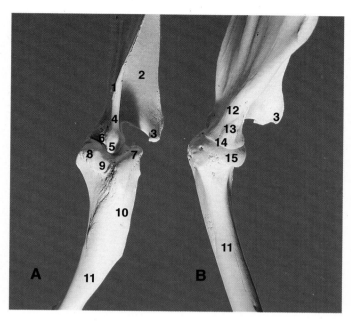

**106 Lateral radiograph of the
shoulder region.** The cranially
advanced limb is the lower limb in
lateral recumbency. To enhance the
outline, the shoulder joint has been
positioned so that its image is
superimposed on that of the
trachea.

1	Seventh cervical vertebra
2	First thoracic vertebra
3	First rib
4	Body of scapula
5	Scapular spine
6	Supraspinatous fossa
7	Infraspinatous fossa
8	Acromion process
9	Trachea
10	Supraglenoid tubercle
11	Infraglenoid tubercle
12	Glenoid cavity
13	Shoulder joint
14	Head of humerus
15	Greater tubercle
16	Body of humerus
17	Deltoid tuberosity
18	Elbow joint
19	Olecranon
20	Sternum
21	Heart
22	Bifurcation of 9
23	Oesophagus (gas filled)

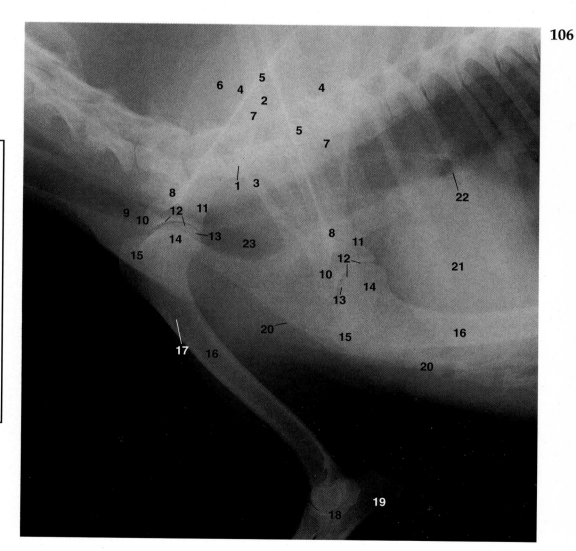

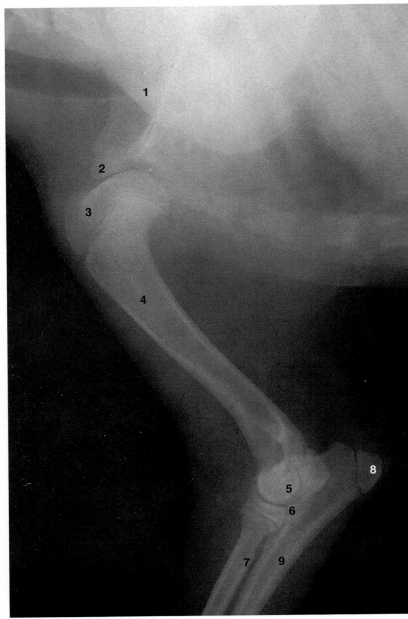

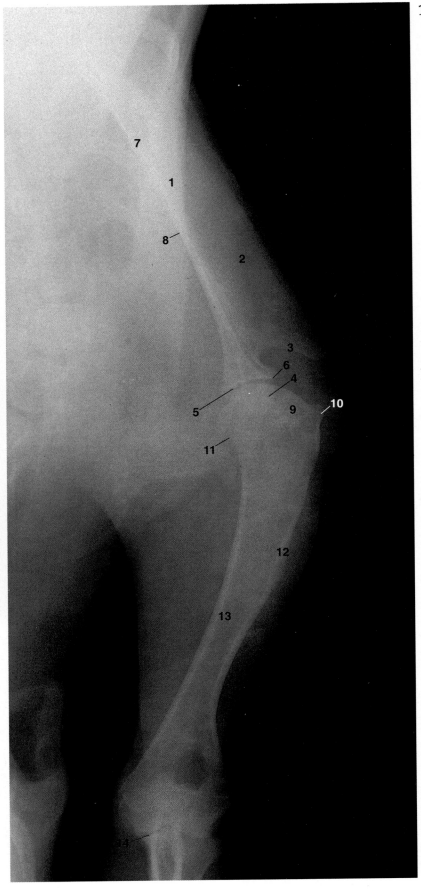

107 Mediolateral radiograph of the shoulder region of a puppy, showing the centres of ossification.

1	Body of scapula
2	Supraglenoid tubercle
3	Proximal humeral epiphysis
4	Body of humerus
5	Distal humeral epiphysis (combined)
6	Proximal radial epiphysis
7	Body of radius
8	Proximal ulnar epiphysis (precursor of olecranon)
9	Body of ulna

108 Caudocranial radiograph of the shoulder joint of a dog.

1	Body ⎫ of scapula
2	Spine ⎭
3	Acromion
4	Supraglenoid tubercle with coracoid process
5	Glenoid cavity
6	Shoulder joint
7	Facies serrata
8	Subscapular fossa
9	Head of humerus
10	Greater tubercle
11	Lesser tubercle
12	Deltoid tuberosity
13	Body of humerus
14	Elbow joint (cubital joint)

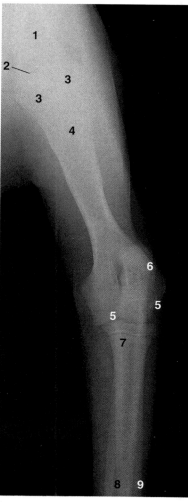

109 Craniocaudal radiograph of the shoulder and brachium of a puppy, showing the centres of ossification.

1	Body of scapula
2	Supraglenoid tubercle
3	Proximal humeral epiphysis
4	Body of humerus
5	Distal humeral epiphysis (combined)
6	Proximal ulnar epiphysis (precursor of olecranon)
7	Proximal radial epiphysis
8	Body of radius
9	Body of ulna

110 Craniocaudal radiograph of the thoracic limb of a kitten, showing the supracondylar foramen.

1	Scapula
2	Suprahamate process
3	Humerus
4	Supratrochlear fossa
5	Supracondylar foramen
6	Radius
7	Ulna
8	Carpus
9	Metacarpals
10	First digit
11	Second to fifth digits

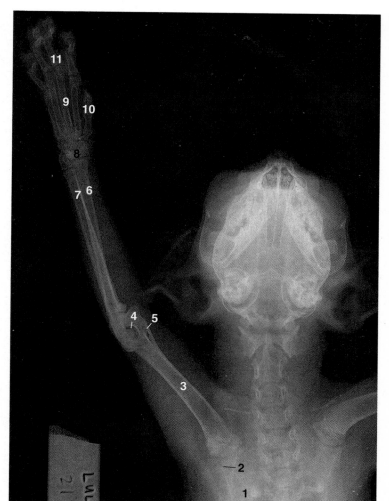

111 Lateral aspect of the superficial muscles of the neck, shoulder, thoracic limb and thoracic wall of a dog.

1	M. trapezius
2	Scapular spine
3	M. cutaneus trunci
4	M. deltoideus
5	Axillobrachial vein
6	M. triceps brachii (long head)
7	M. pectoralis profundus (deep to M. cutaneus trunci)
8	M. triceps brachii (lateral head)
9	Olecranon
10	Extensor group
11	Lateral epicondyle of humerus
12	M. anconeus
13	Superficial brachial artery
14	Radial nerve (superficial lateral and medial branches)
15	Cephalic vein
16	Median cubital vein
17	M. cleidobrachialis
18	M. supraspinatus
19	Greater tubercle of humerus
20	Acromion process
21	Cranial lateral cutaneous nerve (axillary)
22	M. sphincter colli
23	External jugular vein

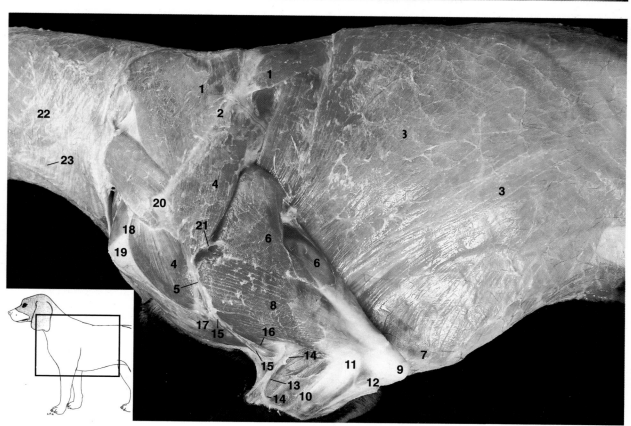

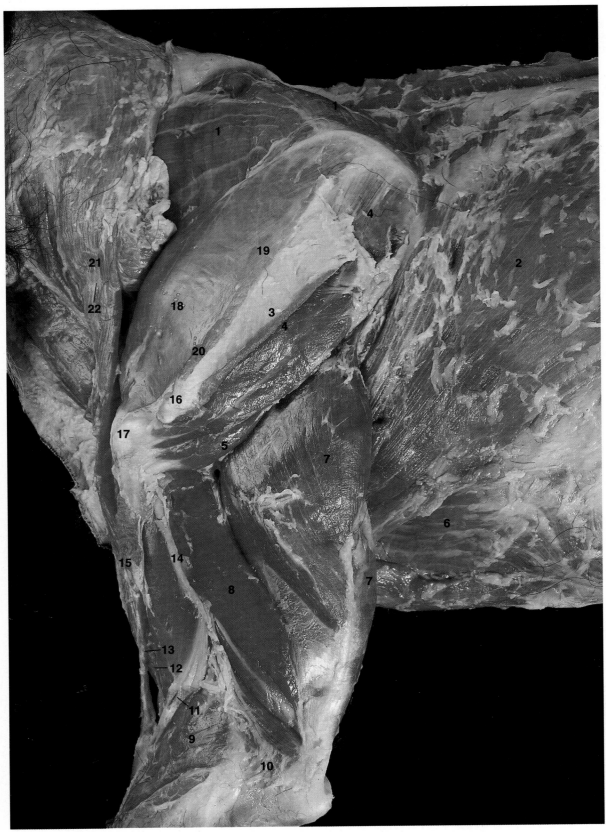

1	M. rhomboideus
2	M. latissimus dorsi
3	M. deltoideus (cut edge)
4	M. infraspinatus
5	M. teres minor
6	M. pectoralis profundus
7	M. triceps brachii (long head)
8	M. triceps brachii (accessory head)
9	M. extensor carpi radialis
10	M. anconeus
11	Radial nerve
12	M. brachialis
13	Cephalic vein
14	Axillobrachial vein
15	M. cleidobrachialis
16	Acromion process
17	Greater tubercle of humerus
18	M. supraspinatus
19	M. trapezius (cut edge)
20	M. omotransversarius (cut edge)
21	M. cleidocephalicus, pars cervicalis
22	Clavicular tendon

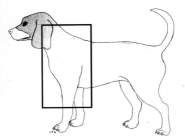

113 Lateral aspect of the deep muscles of the left shoulder and brachium of a dog.
The trapezius and deltoideus muscles have been resected.

1 M. triceps brachii (long head)
2 M. triceps brachii (lateral head)
3 M. triceps brachii (medial head)
4 M. teres minor
5 M. brachialis
6 Radial nerve
7 Medial branch ⎫
8 Lateral branch ⎭ of superficial ramus
9 Deep ramus
10 Muscular branches to triceps
11 M. extensor carpi radialis
12 M. anconeus

- The teres minor muscle crosses the lateral aspect of the shoulder joint. To gain surgical access from a lateral approach, the two heads of the deltoideus are divided to expose the teres minor, which is then rotated from its position or even sectioned to reveal the joint capsule. The radial nerve is seen emerging from its deeper position in the brachial groove. The nerve is vulnerable to trauma in this position, either at the time of a humeral fracture or during reparative surgery.

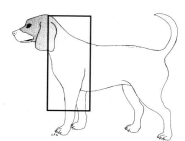

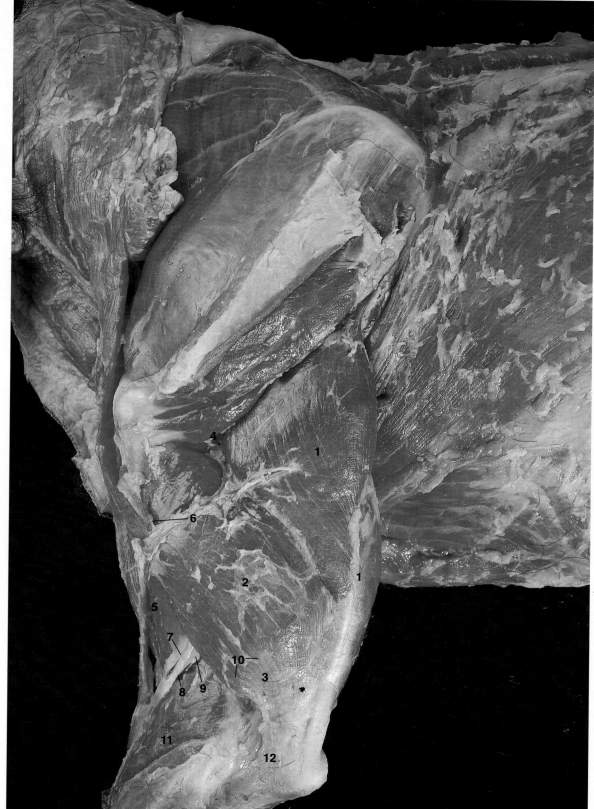

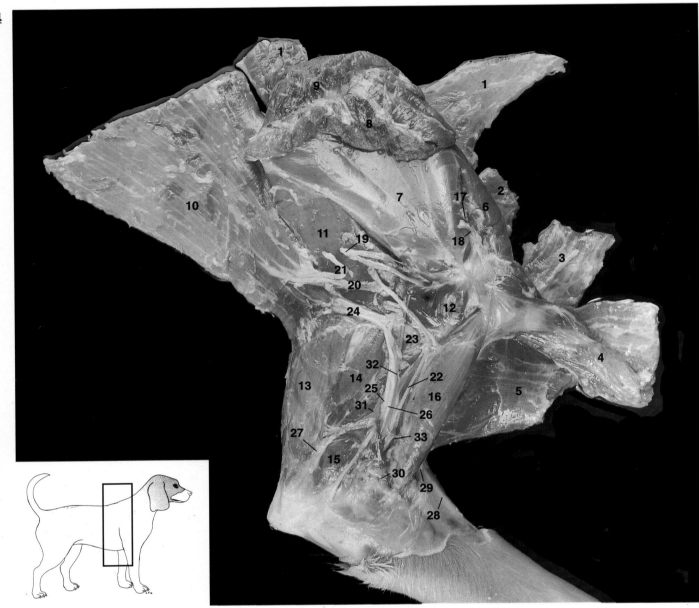

114 Medial aspect of the shoulder and brachium of the detached left thoracic limb of a dog. The extrinsic muscles have been sectioned.

1	M. trapezius	13	M. tensor fasciae antebrachii	25	Ulnar nerve
2	M. omotransversarius	14	M. triceps brachii (long head)	26	Median nerve
3	M. cleidobrachialis with nerve	15	M. triceps brachii (medial head)	27	Caudal cutaneous antebrachial nerve
4	M. pectoralis profundus	16	M. biceps brachii	28	Cephalic vein
5	M. pectorales superficiales	17	Subscapular nerve	29	Median cubital vein
6	M. supraspinatus	18	Suprascapular nerve	30	Median vein
7	M. subscapularis	19	Axillary nerve	31	Brachial vein
8	M. serratus ventralis (cut edge)	20	Lateral thoracic nerve	32	Brachial artery
9	M. rhomboideus (cut edge)	21	Thoracodorsal nerve	33	Bicipital artery
10	M. latissimus dorsi	22	Musculocutaneous nerve		
11	M. teres major	23	Radial nerve		
12	M. coracobrachialis	24	Median and ulnar nerve		

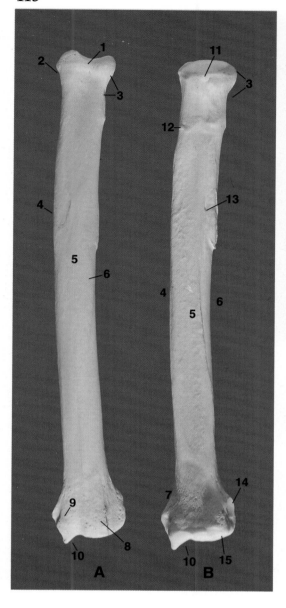

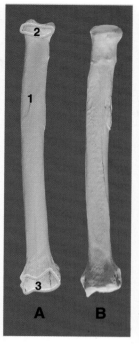

116 Cranial aspect of the left radius (A) and caudal aspect of the right radius (B) of a dog, showing the centres of ossification.

1	Body
2	Proximal
3	Distal

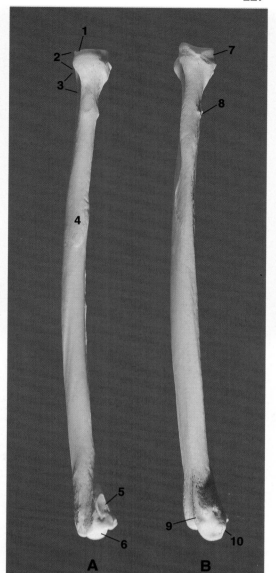

118 Lateral (A) and medial (B) aspect of the radius of a dog, showing areas of muscle attachment.

1	Supinator
2	Pronator teres
3	Abductor pollicis longus
4	Biceps and brachialis
5	Flexor digitorum profundus
6	Pronator quadratus
7	Brachioradialis

115 Cranial aspect of the left radius (A) and caudal aspect of the right radius (B) of a dog.

1	Fovea
2	Head
3	Neck
4	Medial border
5	Body
6	Lateral border
7	Groove for M. extensor digitalis communis
8	Groove for M. extensor carpi radialis
9	Groove for M. abductor pollicis longus
10	Styloid process
11	Articular circumference
12	Radial tuberosity
13	Nutrient foramen
14	Ulnar notch
15	Carpal articular surface

117 Lateral aspect of the left radius (A) and medial aspect of the right radius (B) of a dog.

1	Fovea
2	Head
3	Neck
4	Body
5	Ulnar notch
6	Carpal articular surface
7	Articular circumference
8	Radial tuberosity
9	Grooves for extensor muscles
10	Styloid process

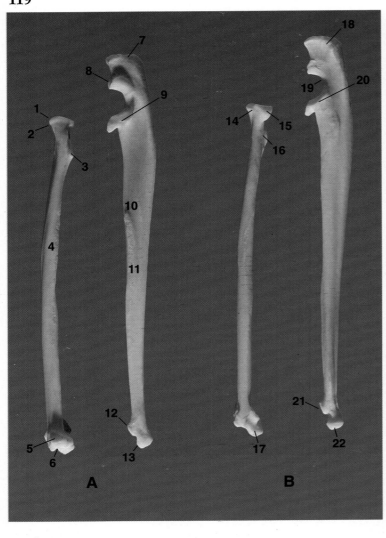

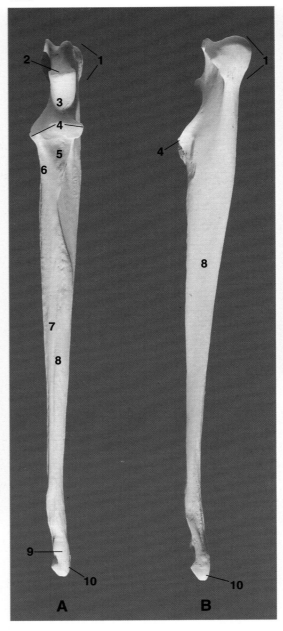

121 Cranial aspect of the left ulna (A) and caudal aspect of the right ulna (B) of a dog, showing centres of ossification.

1	Body
2	Proximal
3	Distal
4	Anconeal (variable)

119 Lateral aspect of the left radius and ulna (A) and medial aspect of the right radius and ulna (B) of a cat.

1	Head ⎫ of radius	12	Ulnar notch
2	Neck ⎭	13	Styloid process of ulna
3	Radial tuberosity	14	Articular circumference
4	Body of radius	15	Articular fovea
5	Ulnar notch	16	Radial tuberosity
6	Carpal articular surface	17	Styloid process of radius
7	Olecranon of ulna	18	Olecranon
8	Anconeal process	19	Trochlear notch
9	Coronoid (lateral) process	20	Coronoid (medial) process
10	Interosseous border	21	Articular circumference
11	Body of ulna	22	Styloid process of ulna

120 Cranial aspect of the left ulna (A) and caudal aspect of the right ulna (B) of a dog.

1	Olecranon
2	Anconeal process
3	Trochlear notch
4	Coronoid process
5	Radial notch
6	Ulnar tuberosity
7	Interosseous border
8	Body
9	Articular circumference
10	Styloid process

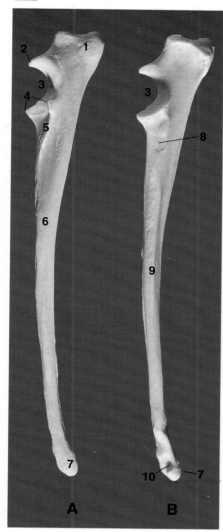

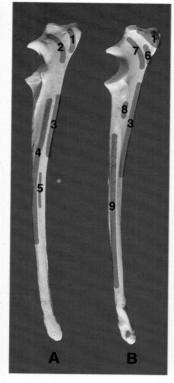

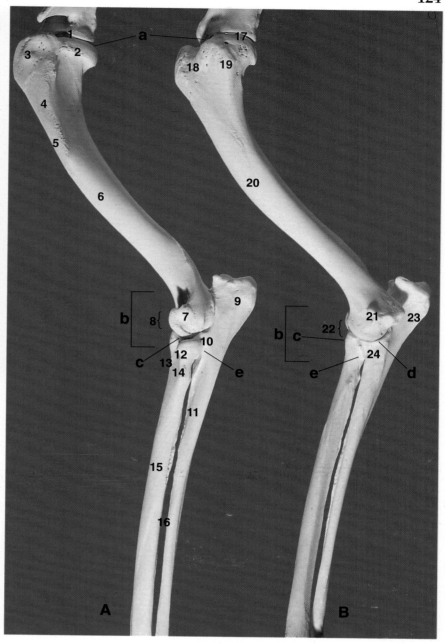

122 Lateral aspect of the left ulna (A) and medial aspect of the right ulna (B) of a dog.

1	Olecranon
2	Anconeal process
3	Trochlear notch
4	Coronoid process
5	Radial notch
6	Body
7	Styloid process
8	Ulnar tuberosity
9	Interosseous border
10	Articular circumference

123 Lateral (A) and medial (B) aspect of the ulna, showing areas of muscle attachment.

1	Triceps
2	Anconeus
3	Flexor digitorum profundus
4	Abductor pollicis longus
5	Extensor pollicis longus
6	Tensor fasciae antebrachii
7	Flexor carpi ulnaris
8	Biceps brachii and brachialis
9	Pronator quadratus

124 Lateral aspect of the left shoulder and elbow joint (A) and medial aspect of the right shoulder and elbow joint (B) of a dog.

a	Shoulder joint	6	Body of humerus
b	Elbow joint (cubital joint)	7	Lateral epicondyle
c	Humeroradial joint	8	Condyle
d	Humero-ulnar joint	9	Olecranon
e	Proximal radio-ulnar joint	10	Coronoid process
		11	Body of ulna
1	Glenoid cavity	12	Fovea
2	Head of humerus	13	Head } of radius
3	Greater tubercle	14	Neck
4	Tricipital line	15	Body
5	Deltoid tuberosity	16	Interosseous space

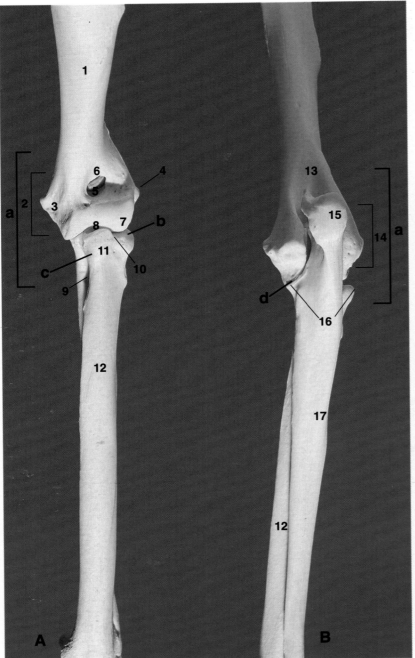

125 Cranial aspect of the left elbow joint (A) and caudal aspect of the right elbow joint (B) of a dog.

126 Craniocaudal radiograph of the elbow of a dog.

a	Elbow joint (cubital joint)	7	Capitulum
b	Humeroradial joint	8	Trochlea
c	Proximal radio-ulnar joint	9	Ulna
d	Humero-ulnar joint	10	Fovea
		11	Head } of radius
1	Body of humerus	12	Body
2	Condyle	13	Olecranon fossa
3	Medial epicondyle	14	Condyle
4	Lateral epicondyle	15	Olecranon
5	Supratrochlear foramen	16	Coronoid process
6	Radial fossa	17	Body of ulna

1	Body of humerus	7	Olecranon fossa
2	Elbow joint (cubital joint)	8	Radius
3	Proximal radio-ulnar joint	9	Ulna
4	Lateral epicondyle	10	Lateral coronoid process
5	Medial epicondyle	11	Medial coronoid process
6	Border of trochlea of humerus	12	Olecranon

127 Mediolateral radiograph of the antebrachium and carpus of a dog.

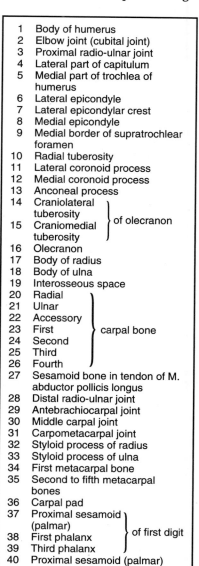

1 Body of humerus
2 Elbow joint (cubital joint)
3 Proximal radio-ulnar joint
4 Lateral part of capitulum
5 Medial part of trochlea of humerus
6 Lateral epicondyle
7 Lateral epicondylar crest
8 Medial epicondyle
9 Medial border of supratrochlear foramen
10 Radial tuberosity
11 Lateral coronoid process
12 Medial coronoid process
13 Anconeal process
14 Craniolateral tuberosity ⎱ of olecranon
15 Craniomedial tuberosity ⎰
16 Olecranon
17 Body of radius
18 Body of ulna
19 Interosseous space
20 Radial ⎫
21 Ulnar |
22 Accessory |
23 First ⎬ carpal bone
24 Second |
25 Third |
26 Fourth ⎭
27 Sesamoid bone in tendon of M. abductor pollicis longus
28 Distal radio-ulnar joint
29 Antebrachiocarpal joint
30 Middle carpal joint
31 Carpometacarpal joint
32 Styloid process of radius
33 Styloid process of ulna
34 First metacarpal bone
35 Second to fifth metacarpal bones
36 Carpal pad
37 Proximal sesamoid ⎫
   (palmar) |
38 First phalanx ⎬ of first digit
39 Third phalanx ⎭
40 Proximal sesamoid (palmar)

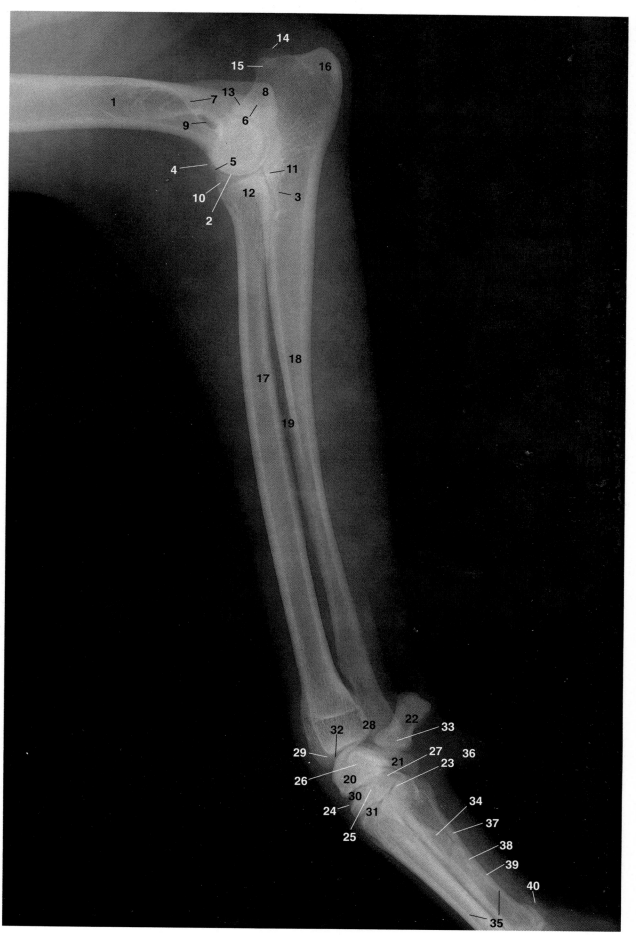

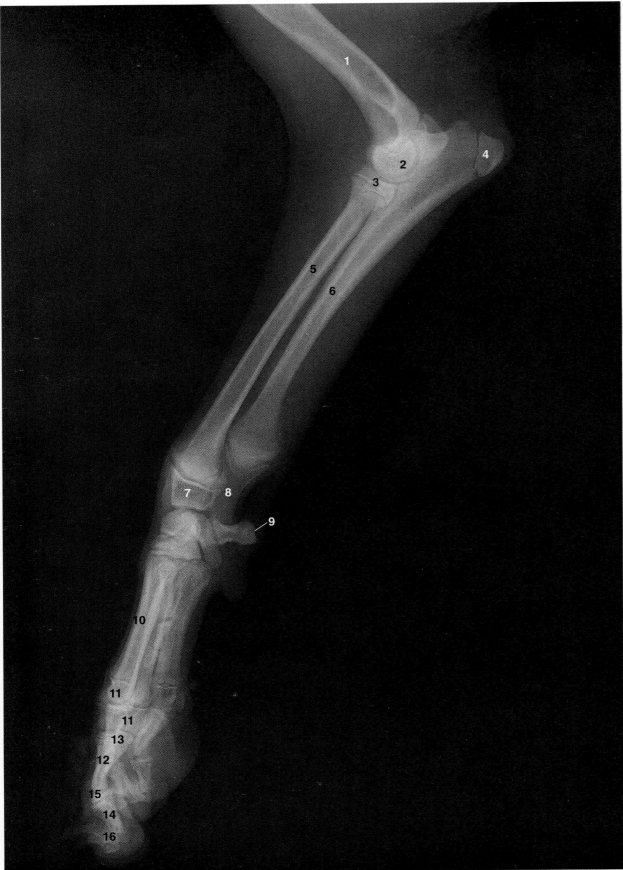

1	Body of humerus
2	Distal humeral epiphysis (combined)
3	Proximal radial epiphysis
4	Proximal ulnar epiphysis (precursor of olecranon)
5	Body of radius
6	Body of ulna
7	Distal radial epiphysis
8	Distal ulnar epiphysis
9	Free epiphysis of accessory carpal bone
10	Body of metacarpus
11	Distal metacarpal epiphysis
12	Body of first phalanx
13	First phalangeal proximal epiphysis
14	Body of second phalanx
15	Second phalangeal proximal epiphysis
16	Body of third phalanx

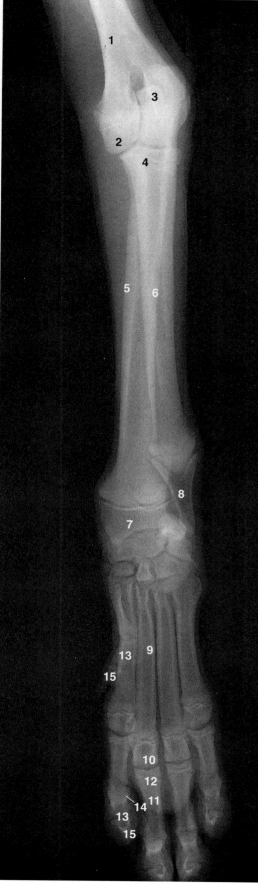

129 Dorsopalmar radiograph of the antebrachium, carpus and manus of a puppy, showing centres of ossification.

1	Body of humerus
2	Distal humeral epiphysis (combined)
3	Proximal ulnar epiphysis (precursor of olecranon)
4	Proximal radial epiphysis
5	Body of radius
6	Body of ulna
7	Distal radial epiphysis
8	Distal ulnar epiphysis
9	Body of metacarpus
10	Distal metacarpal epiphysis
11	Body of first phalanx
12	First phalangeal proximal epiphysis
13	Body of second phalanx
14	Second phalangeal proximal epiphysis
15	Body of third phalanx

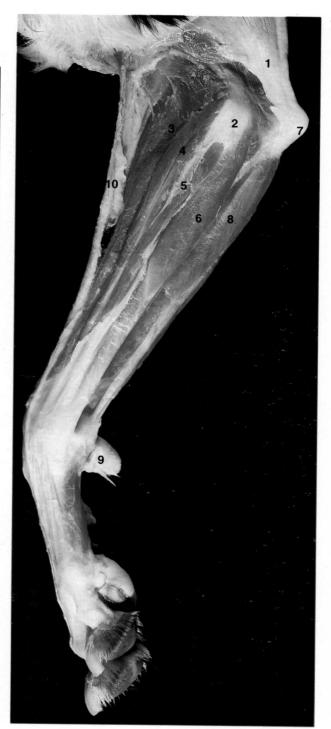

130 Lateral aspect of the antebrachium and manus of the left thoracic limb of a dog.

1	M. triceps brachii
2	Lateral epicondyle of humerus
3	M. extensor carpi radialis
4	M. extensor digitorum communis
5	M. extensor digitorum lateralis
6	M. extensor carpi ulnaris (M. ulnaris lateralis)
7	Olecranon
8	M. flexor carpi ulnaris (ulnar head)
9	Carpal pad
10	Cephalic vein

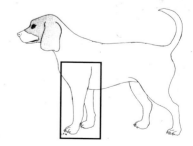

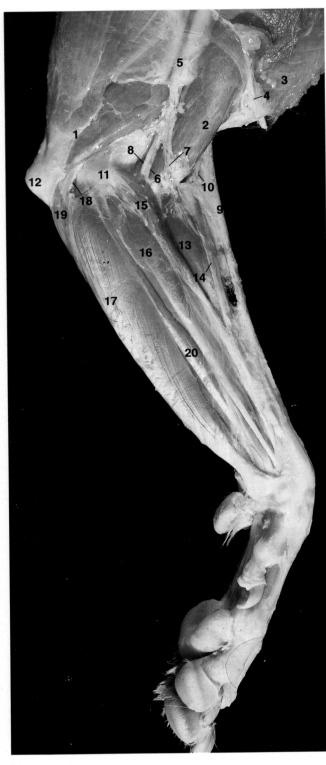

131 Medial aspect of the antebrachium and manus of the left thoracic limb of a dog. The limb has been removed from its attachment to the trunk.

1	M. triceps brachii
2	M. biceps brachii
3	Mm. pectorales superiores
4	Pectoral nerve
5	Brachial vein
6	Brachial artery
7	Superficial radial artery
8	Median nerve
9	Cephalic vein
10	Medial branch of superficial ramus of radial nerve
11	Medial epicondyle of humerus
12	Olecranon
13	M. extensor carpi radialis
14	M. brachioradialis
15	M. pronator teres
16	M. flexor carpi radialis
17	M. flexor digitorum superficialis
18	Ulnar nerve
19	M. flexor carpi ulnaris (ulnar head)
20	M. flexor digitorum profundus (humeral head)

132 Cranial aspect of the antebrachium and dorsal aspect of the manus of the left thoracic limb of a dog.

1	M. extensor carpi radialis
2	M. brachioradialis
3	Cephalic vein
4	Medial and lateral branches of superficial ramus of radial nerve
5	M. extensor digitorum communis
6	M. extensor digitorum lateralis
7	M. abductor pollicis longus
8	Tendon of M. extensor carpi lateralis (M. ulnar lateralis)
9	Tendon of 6
10	Tendon of 5
11	Site of dorsal sesamoid
12	Extensor tendon
13	Accessory cephalic vein
14	Dorsal metacarpal veins
15	Dorsal common digital arteries, veins and nerves

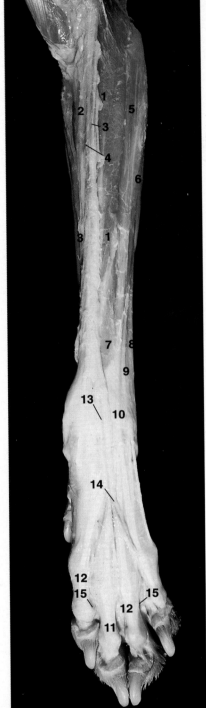

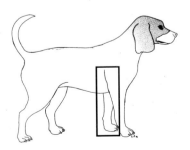

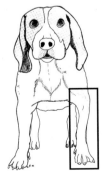

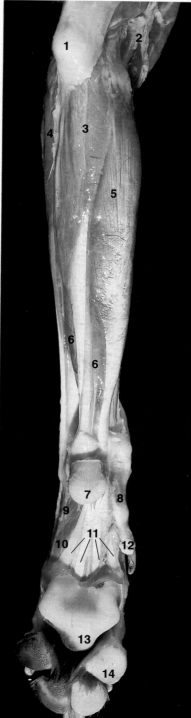

133

134 Dorsal aspect of the left carpus of a dog, in the articulated (A) and the separated (B) form.

1	Radial	
2	Ulnar	
3	Accessory	
4	First	carpal bone
5	Second	
6	Third	
7	Fourth	
8	Articular facet of radius	
9	Lateral process of 2	

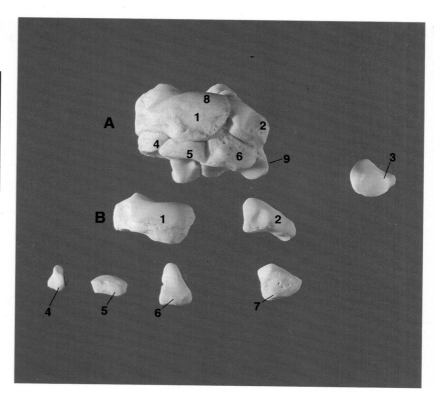

134

135

133 Caudal aspect of the antebrachium and palmar aspect of the manus of the left thoracic limb of a dog. The pads have been left intact.

1	Olecranon	7	Carpal pad
2	Median vessels	8	M. abductor pollicis brevis
3	M. flexor carpi ulnaris (ulnar head)	9	M. abductor digiti quinti
4	M. extensor carpi ulnaris (M. ulnaris lateralis)	10	M. flexor digiti quinti
5	M. flexor digitorum superficialis	11	Tendons of 5
6	M. flexor carpi ulnaris (humeral head)	12	First digit
		13	Metacarpal pad
		14	Digital pads

135 Palmar aspect of the left carpus of a dog, in the articulated (A) and the separated (B) form.

1	Radial	
2	Ulnar	
3	Accessory	
4	First	carpal bone
5	Second	
6	Third	
7	Fourth	
8	Sulcus for tendon of M. flexor carpi radialis	

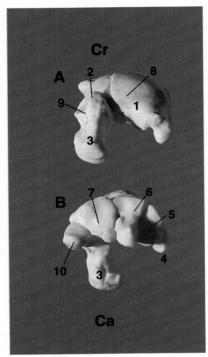

136 Proximal aspect of the left carpus (A) and distal aspect of the right carpus (B) of a dog, oriented cranially (Cr) and caudally (Ca).

1	Radial	
2	Ulnar	
3	Accessory	
4	First	carpal bone
5	Second	
6	Third	
7	Fourth	
8	Articular face for radius	
9	Articular face for ulna	
10	Palmar process of 2	

137

137 Dorsal aspect of the left carpus and manus (A), and palmar aspect of the right carpus and manus (B) of a dog.

a	Carpal joints
b	Antebrachiocarpal joint
c	Middle carpal joint
d	Carpometacarpal joints
e	Intercarpal joints
f	Metacarpophalangeal joints
g	Proximal interphalangeal joint
h	Distal interphalangeal joint

1	Body of ulna	
2	Body of radius	
3	Radial	
4	Ulnar	
5	First	carpal bone
6	Second	
7	Third	
8	Fourth	
9	First metacarpal bone	
10	Second to fifth metacarpal bones	
11	Proximal phalanx	of first digit
12	Distal phalanx	
13	Proximal phalanges	of second to fifth digits
14	Middle phalanges	
15	Distal phalanges	
16	Dorsal sesamoids	
17	Accessory carpal bone	
18	First digit	
19	Palmar sesamoids	

138

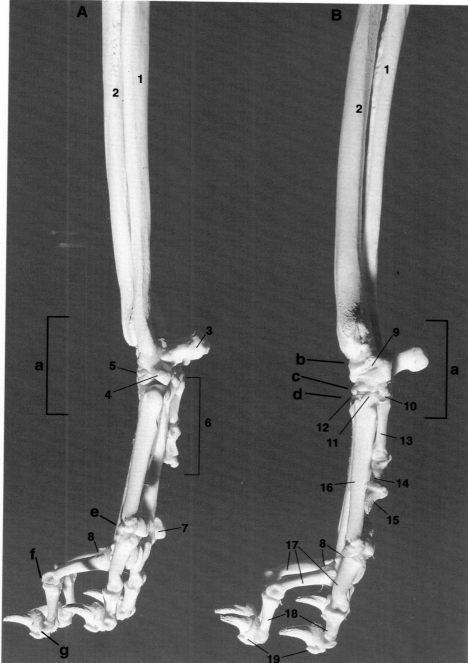

139 Dorsopalmar radiograph of the carpus and manus of a dog.

1	Body of radius
2	Body of ulna
3	Styloid process of radius
4	Styloid process of ulna
5	Distal radio-ulnar joint
6	Antebrachiocarpal joint
7	Radial
8	Ulnar
9	Accessory
10	First } carpal bone
11	Second
12	Third
13	Fourth
14	Middle carpal joint
15	Carpometacarpal joint
16	Sesamoid in the tendon of M. abductor pollicis longus
17	First
18	Second } meta-
19	Third } carpal
20	Fourth } bone
21	Fifth
22	Proximal sesamoids (palmar)
23	Dorsal sesamoid
24	Metacarpophalangeal joint
25	Proximal phalanx of first to fifth digits
26	Proximal interphalangeal joint
27	Middle phalanx of second to fifth digits
28	Distal interphalangeal joint
29	Distal phalanx of first to fifth digits
30	Ungual crest
31	Ungual process

138 Lateral aspect of the left carpus and manus (A), and medial aspect of the right carpus and manus (B) of a dog.

a	Carpal joints	7	Palmar sesamoids
b	Antebrachiocarpal joint	8	Dorsal sesamoids
c	Middle carpal joint	9	Radial
d	Carpometacarpal joints	10	First
e	Metacarpophalangeal joint	11	Second } carpal bone
f	Proximal interphalangeal joint	12	Third
g	Distal interphalangeal joint	13	First metacarpal bone
		14	Proximal phalanx } of first digit
1	Body of ulna	15	Distal phalanx
2	Body of radius	16	Second metacarpal bone
3	Accessory } carpal bone	17	Proximal phalanges } of second
4	Ulnar	18	Middle phalanges } to fifth
5	Fourth	19	Distal phalanges } digits
6	First digit		

139

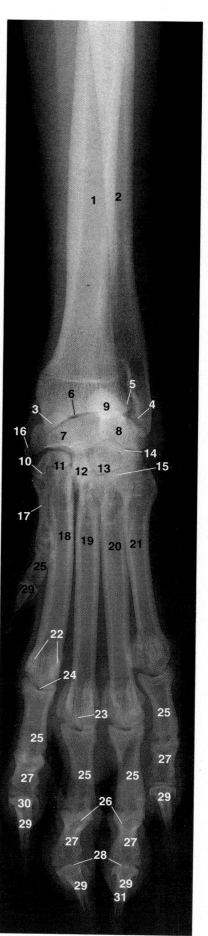

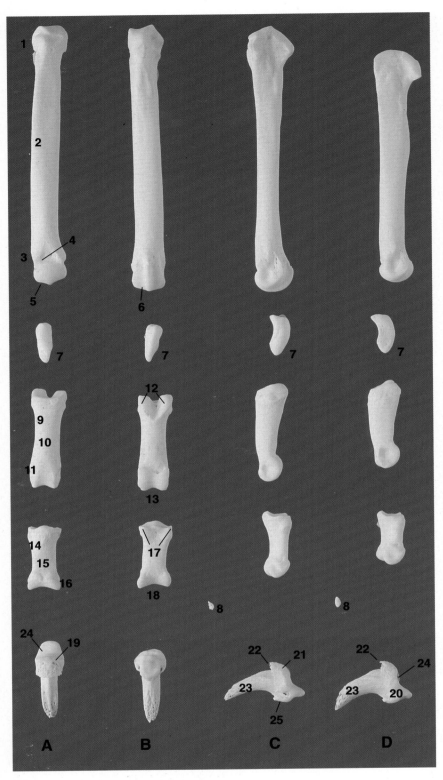

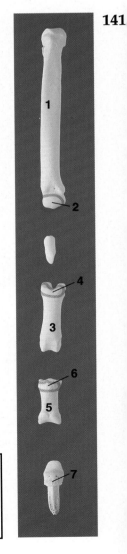

140 Dorsal (A), palmar (B), axial (C) and abaxial (D) aspects of the bones of a typical digit in the manus of a dog.

1	Base	17	Fovea with palmar tubercles and sagittal ridge
2	Body } of metacarpal	18	Trochlea
3	Head	19	Base } of distal phalanx
4	Sesamoid fossa	20	Body
5	Trochlea	21	Extensor tubercle
6	Sesamoid crest	22	Ungual crest
7	Proximal sesamoid	23	Ungual process
8	Dorsal sesamoid	24	Articular surface
9	Base	25	Insertion of M. flexor digitorum profundus
10	Body } of proximal phalanx		
11	Head		
12	Fovea with palmar tubercles		
13	Trochlea		
14	Base		
15	Body } of middle phalanx		
16	Head		

141 Dorsal aspect of a typical digit in the manus of a dog, showing centres of ossification.

1	Body of metacarpus		proximal phalanx
2	Distal metacarpus	5	Body of middle phalanx
3	Body of proximal phalanx	6	Proximal centre of middle phalanx
4	Proximal centre of	7	Body of distal phalanx

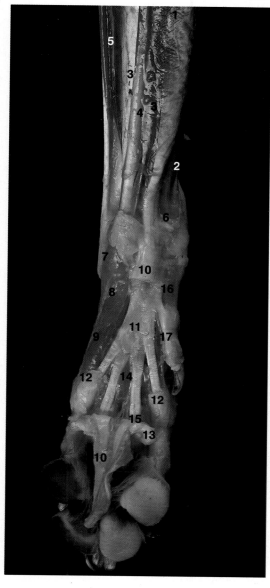

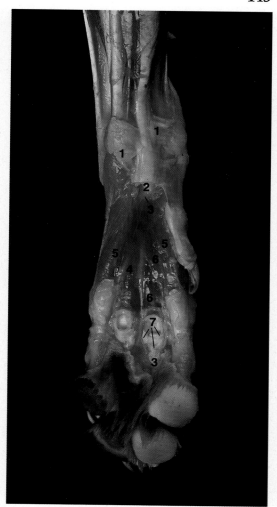

142 Palmar aspect of the manus of the left thoracic limb of a dog. The tendons of the superficial digital flexors have been cut and reflected distally to reveal the deep digital flexor tendons. The carpal and metacarpal pads have been removed.

1	M. flexor digitorum superficialis
2	M. flexor carpi radialis
3	M. flexor carpi ulnaris (humeral head)
4	Tendon of M. flexor carpi ulnaris (ulnar head)
5	M. extensor carpi lateralis (M. ulnaris lateralis)
6	Carpal fascia
7	M. abductor digiti quinti
8	M. flexor digiti quinti
9	Fourth M. interosseus
10	Tendons of 1 (cut)
11	Tendons of M. flexor digitorum profundus
12	Palmar annular ligament
13	Proximal digital annular ligament
14	Mm. lumbricales
15	Position of proximal sesamoids
16	M. abductor pollicis brevis
17	Tendon of M. flexor digitorum profundus to first digit

143 Palmar aspect of the manus of the left thoracic limb of a dog. The tendons of the superficial and deep flexor tendons have been removed to reveal the proximal sesamoids and interosseous muscles.

1	Carpal fascia
2	Tendon of M. flexor digitorum superficialis (cut)
3	Tendon of M. flexor digitorum profundus
4	M. adductor digiti quinti
5	Mm. interossei
6	M. adductor digiti secundi
7	Manica flexoria (tubular sheath of tendon of 2)

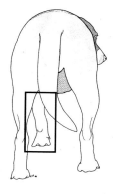

144 Mediolateral radiograph of an arteriogram of the thoracic limb of a dog.

1	Axillary artery
2	Brachial artery
3	Deep brachial artery
4	Bicipital artery
5	Colateral ulnar artery
6	Superficial brachial artery
7	Transverse cubital artery
8	Median artery
9	Recurrent ulnar artery
10	Common interosseous artery
11	Deep antebrachial artery
12	Radial artery
13	Caudal interosseous artery
14	Cranial interosseous artery
15	Ulnar artery
16	Palmar common digital arteries
17	Palmar metacarpal arteries
18	Palmar proper digital arteries

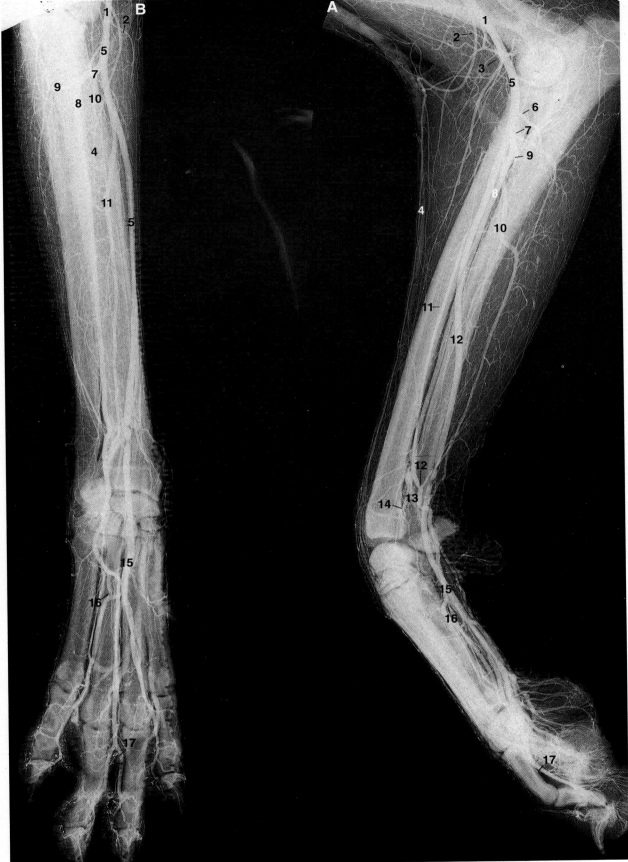

145 Mediolateral (A) and craniocaudal dorsoplantar (B) radiographs of an arteriogram of the thoracic limb of a dog.

1 Brachial artery
2 Superficial brachial artery
3 Transverse cubital artery
4 Cranial superficial antebrachial artery
5 Median artery
6 Recurrent ulnar artery
7 Common interosseous artery
8 Caudal interosseous artery
9 Cranial interosseous artery
10 Ulnar artery
11 Radial artery
12 Anastomosis of the ulnar and caudal interosseous arteries
13 Radial palmar branch
14 Radial dorsal carpal branch
15 Palmar common digital arteries
16 Palmar metacarpal arteries
17 Palmar proper digital arteries
18 Dorsal proper digital arteries

146 Mediolateral radiograph of a venogram of the thoracic limb of a dog.

1   Accessory cephalic vein
2   Cephalic vein
3   Radial vein
4   Interosseous vein
5   Ulnar vein
6   Median vein
7   Median cubital vein
8   Brachial vein
9   Axillobrachial vein
10 Omobrachial vein
11 Axillary vein
12 External jugular vein
13 Internal thoracic vein
14 Precava
15 Cranial vena cava
16 Right side of heart

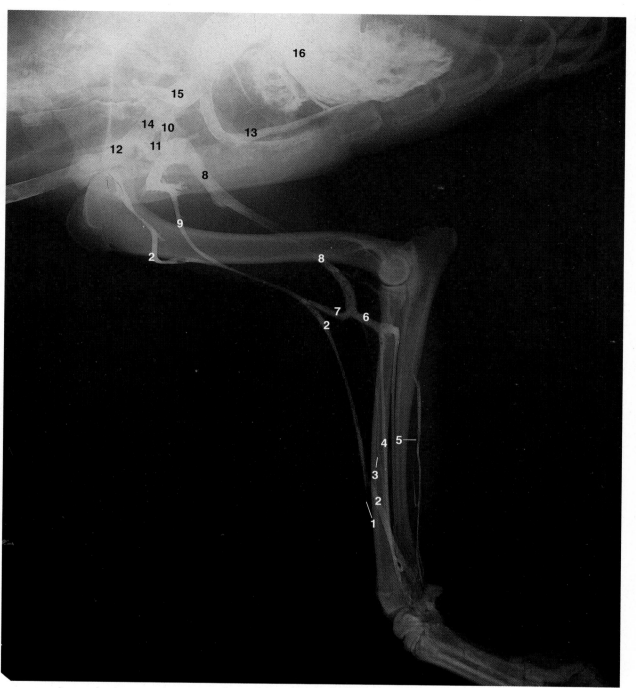

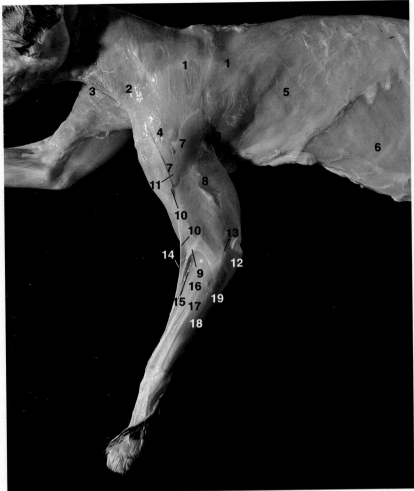

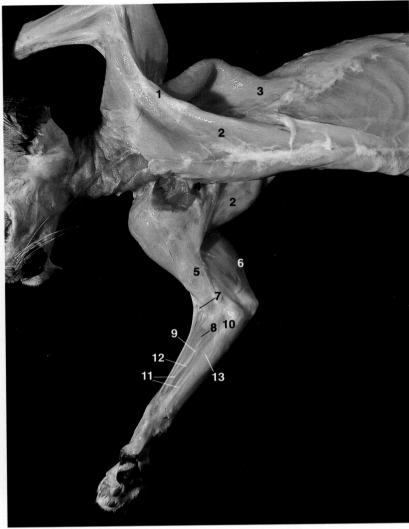

147 Lateral aspect of the superficial muscles of the left thoracic limb of a cat.

1	M. trapezius	11	Omobrachial vein
2	M. brachiocephalicus	12	Olecranon
3	M. sternocephalicus	13	M. anconeus
4	M. omotransversarius	14	M. brachioradialis
5	M. latissimus dorsi	15	M. extensor carpi radialis
6	M. obliquus externus abdominis	16	M. extensor digitorum communis
7	M. deltoideus	17	M. extensor digitorum lateralis
8	M. triceps brachii	18	M. extensor carpi ulnaris (M.
9	Radial nerve		ulnaris lateralis)
10	Cephalic vein	19	M. flexor carpi ulnaris

148 Medial aspect of the superficial muscles of the left thoracic limb of a cat.

1	Mm. pectorales superficiales	7	Cephalic vein
2	M. pectoralis profundus	8	M. brachioradialis
3	M. latissimus dorsi	9	M. extensor carpi radialis
4	Axillary space exposed by	10	M. pronator teres
	sectioning of 1 and 2	11	M. flexor digitorum profundus
5	M. biceps brachii	12	M. flexor carpi radialis
6	M. triceps brachii	13	M. flexor digitorum superficialis

5 Thorax

The osteological features of the thoracic region are revealed using bony specimens and radiographs. With prepared dissections, the musculature is serially displayed from the superficial to the deep layers to reveal the thoracic contents and to demonstrate the topography. The additional technique of B-mode ultrasonography is used to further illustrate cardiac anatomy, and cross-sectional specimens tie together the topographical relationships of the intrathoracic organs.

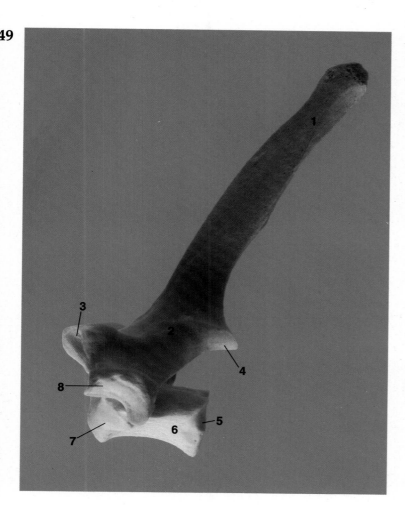

149 Lateral aspect of the first thoracic vertebra of a dog.

1	Spinous process	6	Body
2	Lamina	7	Cranial costal fovea
3	Mamillary process	8	Costal fovea of transverse
4	Caudal articular surface		process
5	Caudal costal fovea		

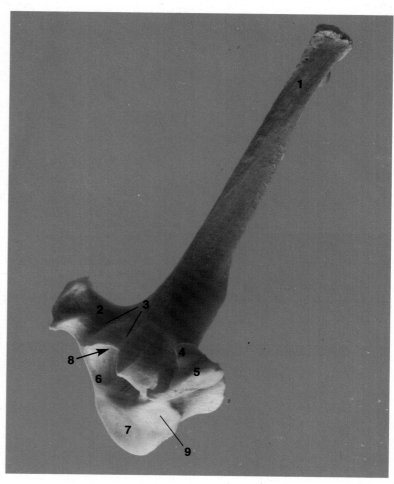

150 Craniolateral aspect of the sixth thoracic vertebra of a dog.

1	Spinous process	6	Pedicle
2	Lamina	7	Body
3	Cranial articular surface	8	Vertebral foramen
4	Transverse process	9	Cranial costal fovea
5	Costal fovea of 4		

151

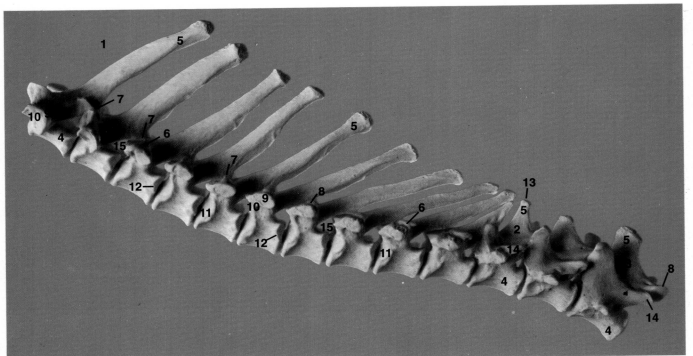

1	First		6	Cranial articular process	11	Cranial costal fovea
2	Eleventh	} thoracic vertebra	7	Mamillary process	12	Caudal costal fovea
3	Thirteenth		8	Caudal articular process	13	Anticlinal vertebra
4	Body		9	Transverse process	14	Accessory process
5	Spinous process		10	Cranial costal fovea of 9	15	Intervertebral foramen

152

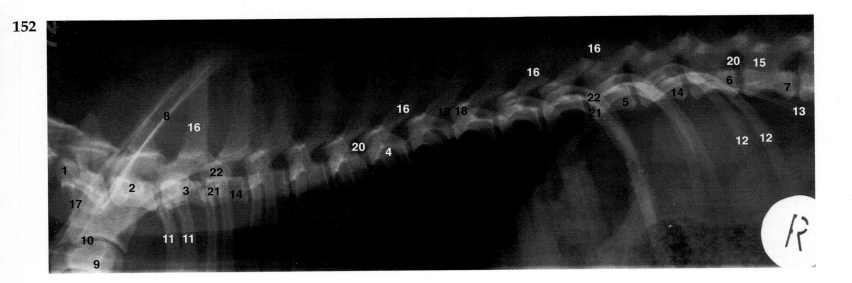

152 Radiograph of the lateral aspect of the thoracic portion of the vertebral column of a dog.

1	Sixth	} cervical vertebra	9	Humerus	16	Spinous process
2	Seventh		10	Shoulder joint	17	Transverse process (plate-like lamina of sixth cervical vertebra)
3	First		11	First	} rib		
4	Sixth	} thoracic vertebra	12	Twelfth		18	Cranial articular process
5	Eleventh (anticlinal)		13	Thirteenth (floating)		19	Caudal articular process
6	Thirteenth		14	Body		20	Intervertebral foramina
7	First lumbar vertebra		15	Dorsal and ventral borders of vertebral foramen (vertebral canal)	21	Head	} of rib
8	Scapula				22	Tubercle	

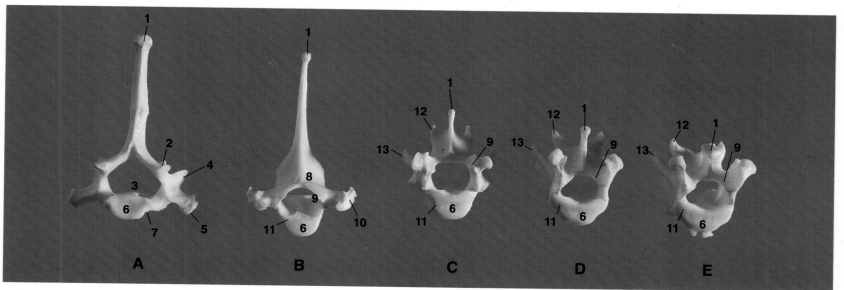

153 Caudal aspect of the first thoracic vertebra (A) and cranial aspect of the sixth (B), eleventh (C), twelfth (D) and thirteenth (E) thoracic vertebrae of a cat.

1	Spinous process	7	Caudal costal fovea
2	Caudal articular surface	8	Lamina
3	Vertebral foramen	9	Cranial articular surface
4	Mamillary process	10	Transverse process
5	Transverse process (with cranial costal fovea)	11	Cranial costal fovea
		12	Caudal articular process
6	Body	13	Accesory process

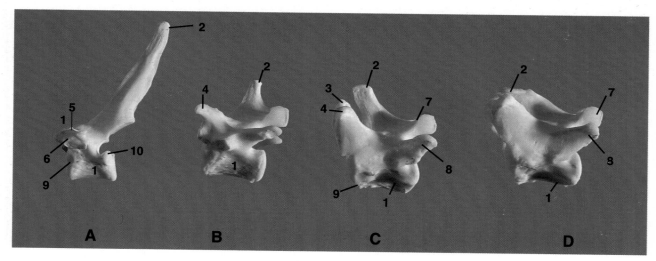

154 Left lateral aspect of the sixth (A), eleventh (anticlinal) (B), twelfth (C) and thirteenth (D) thoracic vertebrae of a cat.

1	Body	6	Costal fovea of 5
2	Spinous process	7	Caudal articular process
3	Cranial articular process	8	Accessory process
4	Mamillary process	9	Cranial costal fovea
5	Transverse process	10	Caudal costal fovea

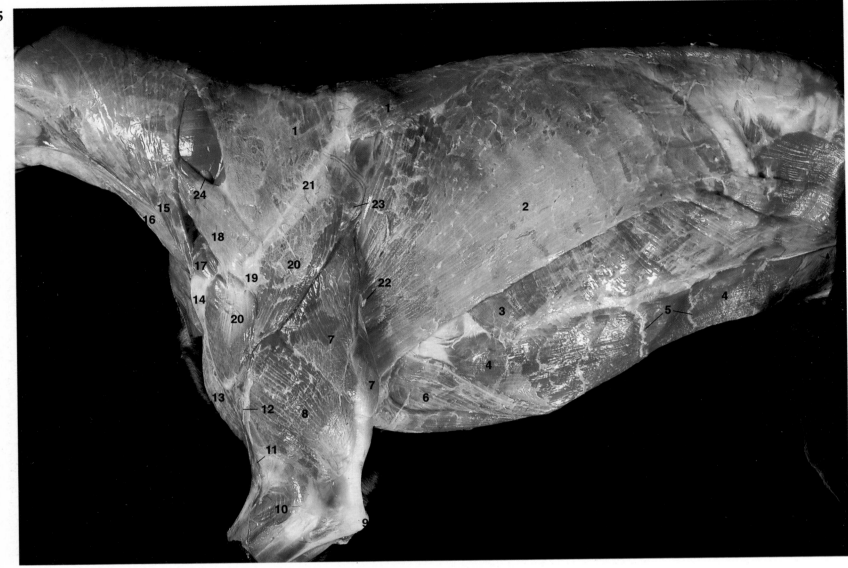

155 Lateral aspect of the superficial muscles of the shoulder and brachium of a dog. The cutaneous trunci and sphincter colli muscles have been removed.

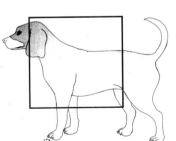

1	M. trapezius	10	Extensor group	18	M. omotransversarius
2	M. latissimus dorsi	11	Cephalic vein	19	Acromion process
3	M. obliquus externus abdominis	12	Axillobrachial vein	20	M. deltoideus
4	M. rectus abdominis	13	M. cleidobrachialis	21	Scapular spine
5	Tendinous intersections	14	Greater tubercle of humerus	22	Intercostobrachial nerve (second thoracic nerve)
6	M. pectoralis profundus	15	M. cleidocephalicus, pars cervicalis	23	Subscapular artery and vein
7	M. triceps brachii (long head)	16	M. sternocephalicus	24	Superficial cervical lymph nodes
8	M. triceps brachii (lateral head)	17	M. supraspinatus		
9	Olecranon				

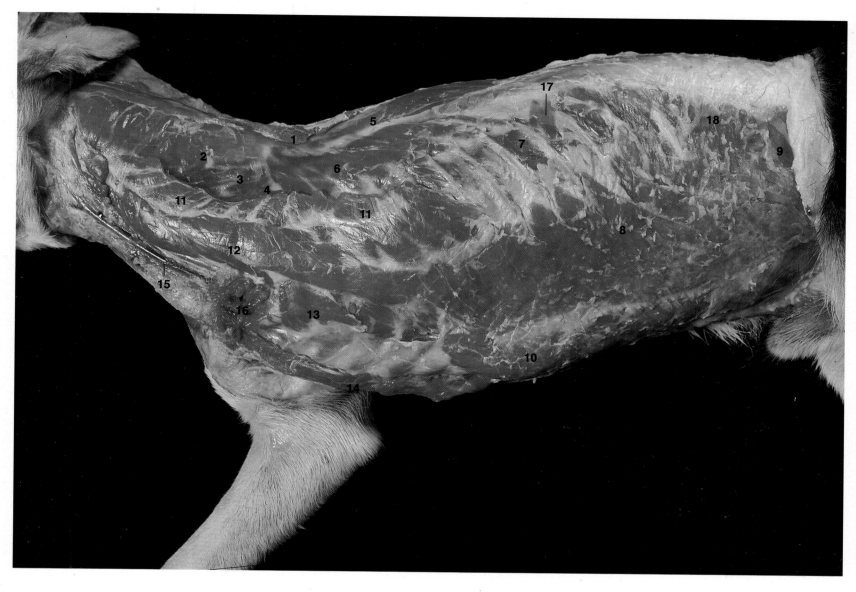

156 Lateral aspect of the muscles of the neck, thorax and abdominal wall of a dog. The left thoracic limb has been removed along with its extrinsic muscles. The axillary vessels and the brachial plexus have been sectioned in the process.

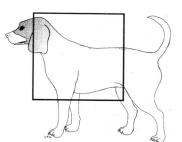

1	M. rhomboideus (cut)	8	M. obliquus externus abdominis, pars costalis	14	Mm. pectorales (cut)
2	M. splenius			15	External jugular vein
3	M. longissimus cervicis	9	M. obliquus externus abdominis, pars lumbalis	16	Axillary vessels (cut)
4	M. longissimus thoracis			17	M. serratus dorsalis caudalis
5	M. spinalis and M. semispinalis thoracis	10	M. rectus abdominis	18	M. obliquus internus abdominis, pars costalis
6	M. serratus dorsalis cranialis	11	M. serratus ventralis (cut)		
7	Mm. intercostales	12	M. scalenus		
		13	M. rectus thoracis		

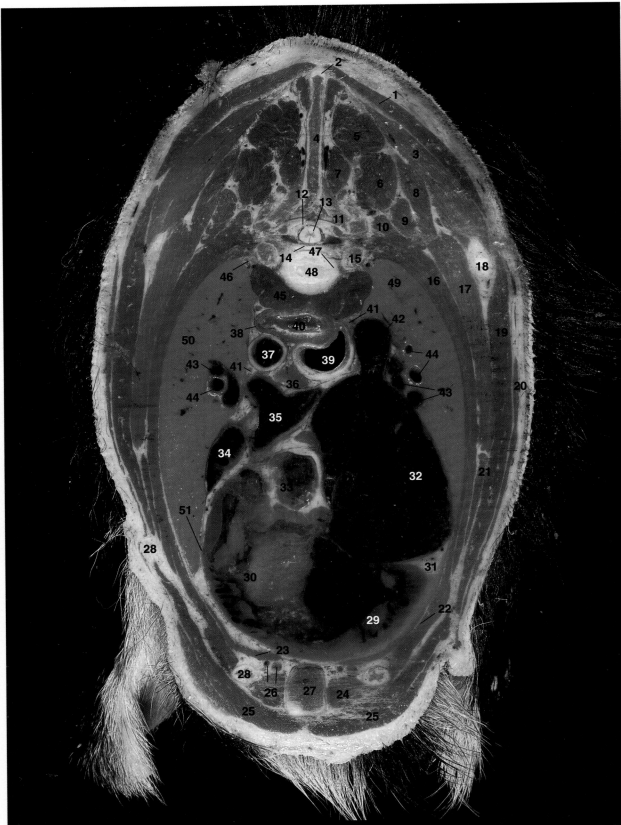

1	M. trapezius
2	Supraspinous ligament
3	M. rhomboideus
4	Spinous process of fourth thoracic vertebra
5	M. spinalis and m. semispinalis (thoracis and cervicalis)
6	M. longissimus thoracis
7	M. multifidus thoracis
8	M. serratus dorsalis cranialis
9	M. iliocostalis thoracis
10	Mm. rotatores
11	Arch of fourth thoracic vertebra
12	Epidural fat
13	Spinal cord
14	Intercapital ligament
15	Head of rib (caput)
16	Mm. intercostales externi and interni
17	M. serratus ventralis
18	Scapula
19	M. latissimus dorsi
20	M. cutaneus trunci
21	M. scalenus
22	M. rectus abdominis
23	M. transversus thoracis
24	M. intercostalis internus
25	M. pectoralis profundus
26	Internal thoracic artery and vein
27	Sternum
28	Costal cartilage
29	Right ventricle
30	Left ventricle
31	Pericardium overlying coronary vessels in fat of coronary groove
32	Right atrium
33	Left ventricular outflow tract (aortic valve)
34	Left auricle
35	Pulmonary artery (bifurcating)
36	Tracheobronchial lymph node
37	Aorta
38	Thoracic duct
39	Trachea
40	Oesophagus
41	Left and right vagus nerves
42	Right azygos vein
43	Pulmonary veins
44	Bronchi
45	M. longus colli
46	Sympathetic trunk
47	Annulus fibrosus } of intervertebral disc
48	Nucleus pulposus }
49	Cranial lobe of right lung
50	Cranial lobe of left lung
51	Phrenic nerve

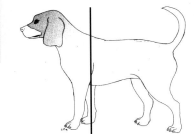

158 Lateral aspect of the left thorax of a dog. The muscles of the thoracic wall and thoracic limb have been resected, along with alternate ribs.

1	M. serratus dorsalis cranialis
2	Brachial plexus
3	Axillary vessels
4	First
5	Fifth
6	Ninth
7	Thirteenth (floating)
8	Pars sternalis
9	Pars costalis
10	Centrum tendineum
11	Left costodiaphragmatic recess
12	M. obliquus externus abdominis
13	Heart
14	Mediastinal pleura
15	Caudal lobe
16	Caudal part of cranial lobe
17	Cranial part of cranial lobe
18	Thymus
19	Costochondral joints
20	Costal cartilages
21	Sternum
22	Costal arch

(4, 5, 6, 7 — rib; 8, 9, 10 — of diaphragm; 16, 17 — of left lung)

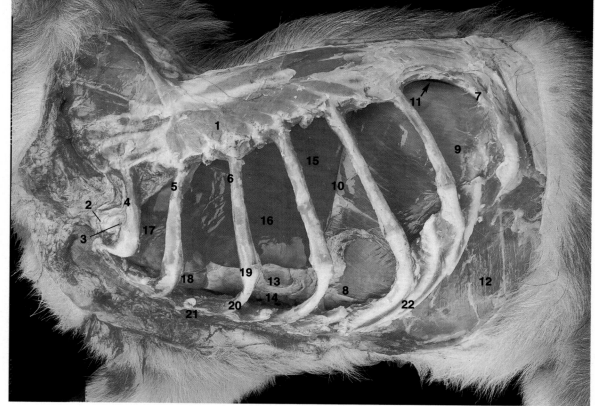

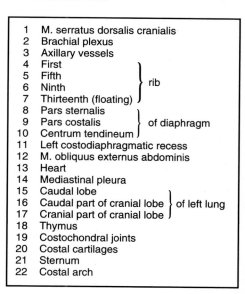

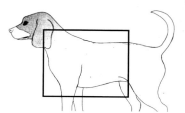

159 Lateral aspect of the opened right thorax of a dog. The right thoracic wall and thoracic limb have been removed, along with alternate ribs.

1	Brachial plexus
2	Intercostal vessels
3	First
4	Fourth
5	Eighth
6	Thirteenth (floating)
7	Right costodiaphragmatic recess
8	M. obliquus externus abdominis
9	M. obliquus internus abdominis
10	Pars costalis
11	Pars sternalis
12	Caudal lobe
13	Middle lobe
14	Cranial lobe
15	Cardiac notch
16	Heart
17	Mediastinal pleura
18	Sternum

(3, 4, 5, 6 — rib; 10, 11 — of diaphragm; 12, 13, 14 — of right lung)

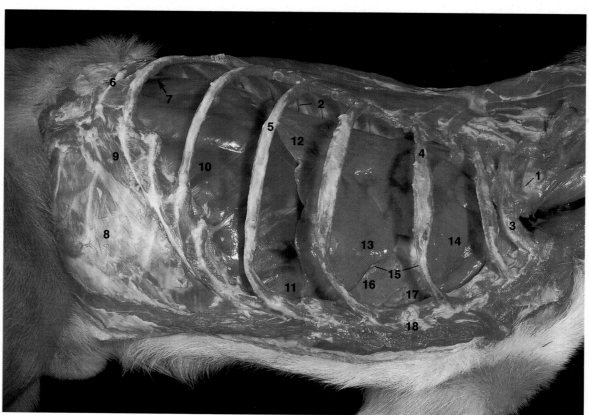

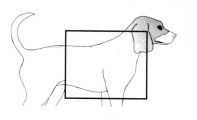

160

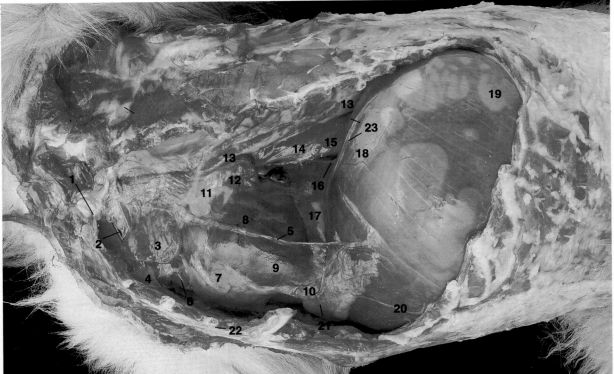

1	Brachial plexus
2	Internal thoracic vein and artery
3	Thymus
4	Mediastinal pleura
5	Phrenic nerve
6	Right auricle
7	Right ventricle
8	Left auricle
9	Left ventricle
10	Apex } of heart
11	Base } of heart
12	Pulmonary (cut) vessels and left bronchus
13	Aorta
14	Oesophagus
15	Dorsal branch } of vagus nerve
16	Ventral branch } of vagus nerve
17	Accessory lobe of right lung
18	Centrum tendineum
19	Pars costalis } of diaphragm
20	Pars sternalis } of diaphragm
21	Position of sternopericardiac ligament
22	Fifth rib and costal cartilage
23	Hiatus oesophageus

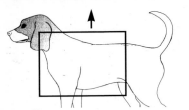
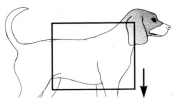

161

161 Lateral aspect of the opened right thorax of a dog. The right lung has been resected to expose the mediastinum and its contents.

1	First rib
2	Brachial plexus
3	Internal thoracic artery and vein
4	Right costocervical vein
5	Cranial vena cava
6	Vagus nerve (crossing trachea)
7	Right azygos vein
8	Cranial lobe of left lung
9	Thymus
10	Mediastinal pleura
11	Right phrenic nerve
12	Base of heart
13	Right ventricle
14	Right atrium
15	Left ventricle
16	Fifth rib
17	Pulmonary vessels (cut) and bronchus
18	Oesophagus with vagus nerve
19	Left lung
20	Plica venae cavae
21	Apex of heart
22	Pars sternalis } of diaphragm
23	Centrum tendineum } of diaphragm
24	Pars costalis } of diaphragm
25	Foramen venae cavae
26	Caudal vena cava
27	Thirteenth (floating) rib

162 Ventral aspect of the opened thorax of a dog. The sternum and costal cartilages have been removed to reveal the thoracic viscera.

1 Larynx with M. cricothyroideus
2 Trachea
3 Thyroid gland
4 M. sternothyroideus
5 M. sternicephalicus
6 Carotid sheath (containing common carotid artery and vagosympathetic trunk)
7 External jugular vein
8 Manubrium sterni
9 Axillary vessels
10 Mediastinal pleura
11 Cranial vena cava
12 Right azygos vein
13 Cranial lobe ⎫
14 Middle lobe ⎬ of right lung
15 Caudal lobe ⎪
16 Accessory lobe ⎭
17 Cranial part of left lobe ⎫ of left lung
18 Caudal part of left lobe ⎬
19 Caudal lobe ⎭
20 Right subclavian artery
21 Left subclavian artery
22 Right atrium
23 Base of heart
24 Right ventricle
25 Pericardium
26 Pulmonary vessels at hilus of lung
27 Caudal vena cava with right phrenic nerve
28 Pars sternalis ⎫ of
29 Centrum tendineum ⎬ diaphragm
30 Foramen venae cavae
31 Xiphoid process
32 Left ventricle
33 Apex of heart

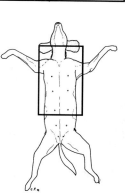

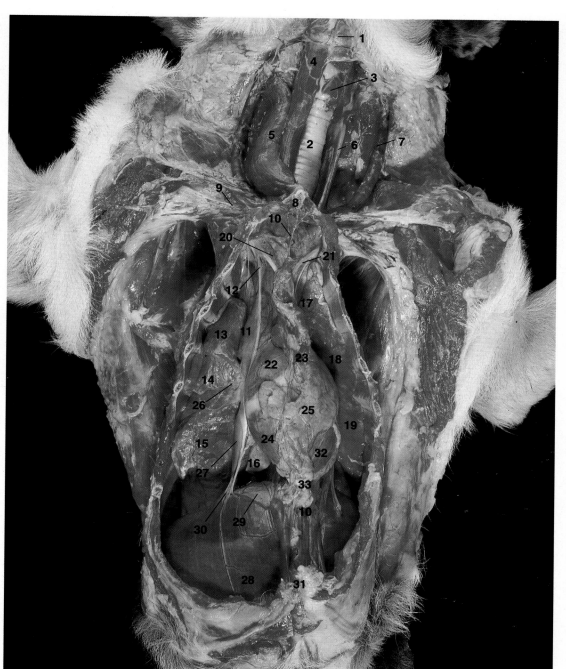

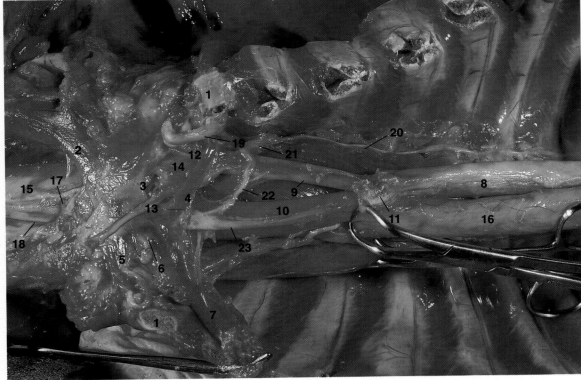

163 Exposure of the dorsocranial region of the thorax of a dog. The thoracic viscera have been resected by severing the aortic arch and the venae cavae at the base of the base of the heart.

1	First rib
2	Left brachiocephalic vein
3	Left subclavian vein
4	Left costocervical vein
5	Right brachiocephalic vein
6	Internal thoracic vein (cut)
7	Cranial vena cava (cut with artery forceps)
8	Descending aorta
9	Left subclavian artery
10	Brachiocephalic artery
11	Proximal end of aortic arch (cut)
12	Costocervical trunk
13	Internal thoracic artery
14	Continuation of subclavian artery to become axillary artery
15	Cervical oesophagus
16	Thoracic oesophagus
17	Recurrent laryngeal nerve
18	Carotid sheath (containing common carotid artery and vagosympathetic trunk)
19	Vertebral nerve
20	Sympathetic trunk or chain
21	Cervicothoracic ganglion (stellate)
22	Ansa subclavia
23	Left vagus nerve (cut)

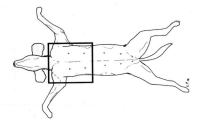

164 Cranial aspect of the diaphragm of a dog, viewed from the right. The lungs have been removed and the heart displaced caudally.

1	Apex of heart
2	Cranial vena cava
3	Sympathetic trunk
4	Caudal vena cava
5	Foramen venae cavae
6	Oesophagus
7	Hiatus oesophageus
8	Vagus nerve
9	Aorta
10	Hiatus aorticus
11	Pars costalis
12	Pars sternalis
13	Pars lumbalis
14	Centrum tendineum
15	Xiphoid process
16	Recessus phrenicolumbalis
17	M. serratus ventralis

(11–14: of diaphragm)

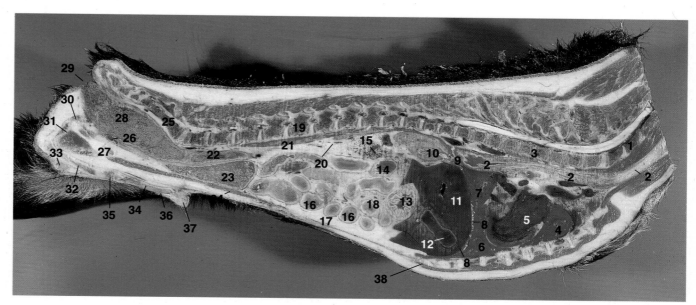

165 Paramedian section through the thoracic, abdominal and pelvic cavities of a male dog, showing the topography of the structures of the left side.

1	Cervical vertebrae	20	Aorta
2	Oesophagus	21	M. psoas major
3	Thoracic vertebrae	22	Descending colon
4	Cranial lobe of left lung	23	Urinary bladder
5	Right ventricle	24	M. rectus abdominis
6	Accessory lobe of right lung	25	Sacrum
7	Caudal lobe of left lung	26	Prostate
8	Diaphragm	27	Symphysis pelvis
9	Hiatus oesophageus	28	Rectum
10	Cardiac region of stomach	29	Anus
11	Liver	30	Root of penis
12	Gall bladder	31	Corpus cavernosum penis
13	Pyloric region of stomach	32	Body of penis
14	Transverse colon	33	Testis
15	Pancreas	34	Glans penis
16	Jejunum	35	Bulbus glandis
17	Greater omentum	36	Pars longa glandis
18	Great mesentery	37	Prepuce
19	Lumbar vertebrae	38	Xiphoid process of sternum

166 Paramedian section through the thoracic, abdominal and pelvic cavities of a male dog, showing the topography of the structures of the right side.

1	Cervical vertebrae	12	Stomach
2	Spinal cord	13	Lumbar vertebrae
3	Trachea	14	Mesenteric lymph node
4	Thoracic vertebrae	15	Transverse duodenum
5	Manubrium sterni	16	Urinary bladder
6	Oeosphagus	17	Descending colon
7	Cranial vena cava	18	Rectum
8	Right ventricle	19	Sacrum
9	Diaphragm	20	Caudal vertebrae
10	Liver	21	Symphysis of pubis
11	Gall bladder		

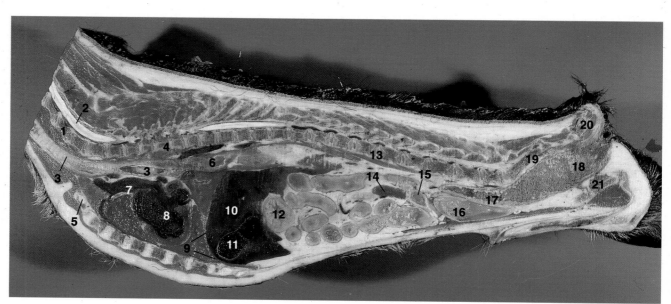

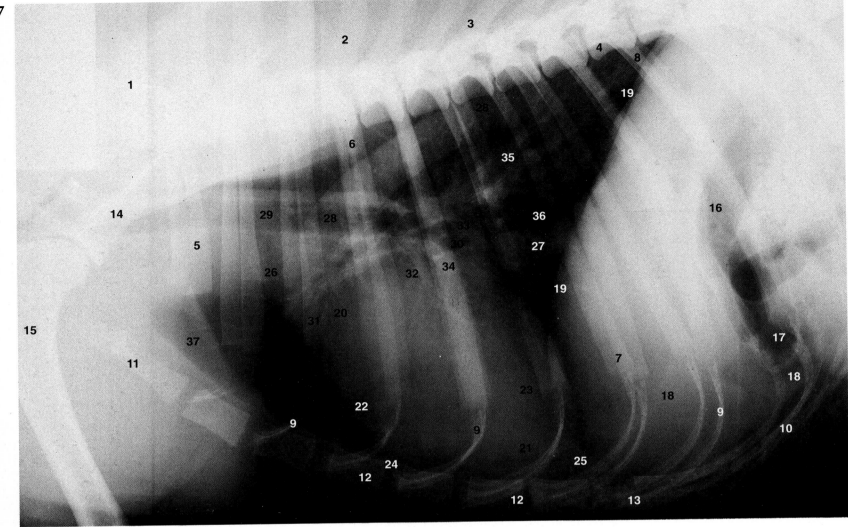

167 Radiograph of the thoracic region of a dog in lateral recumbency.

1	First ⎫		14	Scapula
2	Fourth ⎬ thoracic vertebra		15	Humerus
3	Seventh ⎪		16	Stomach
4	Tenth ⎭		17	Small intestine
5	First ⎫		18	Liver
6	Fourth ⎬ rib		19	Diaphragm
7	Seventh ⎪		20	Base ⎫
8	Tenth ⎭		21	Apex ⎬ of heart
9	Costal cartilage		22	Right side ⎪
10	Costal arch		23	Left side ⎭
11	Manubrium sterni		24	Pericardium
12	Sternebrae		25	Sternopericardiac ligament
13	Xiphoid process		26	Cranial vena cava

27 Caudal vena cava
28 Aorta
29 Trachea
30 Tracheal bifurcation
31 Bronchus to cranial ⎫
32 Bronchus to middle ⎬ lobe of lung
33 Bronchus to caudal ⎭
34 Bronchus to accessory lobe of right lung
35 Dorsal bronchi
36 Ventral bronchi
37 Pleural cupula

168 Ventrodorsal radiograph of the thoracic region of a dog.

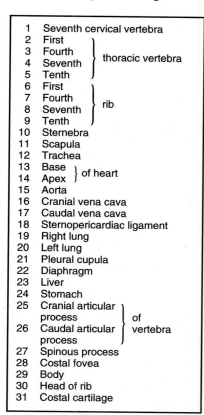

1 Seventh cervical vertebra
2 First ⎫
3 Fourth ⎬ thoracic vertebra
4 Seventh ⎪
5 Tenth ⎭
6 First ⎫
7 Fourth ⎬ rib
8 Seventh ⎪
9 Tenth ⎭
10 Sternebra
11 Scapula
12 Trachea
13 Base ⎫ of heart
14 Apex ⎬
15 Aorta
16 Cranial vena cava
17 Caudal vena cava
18 Sternopericardiac ligament
19 Right lung
20 Left lung
21 Pleural cupula
22 Diaphragm
23 Liver
24 Stomach
25 Cranial articular ⎫ of
   process ⎬ vertebra
26 Caudal articular ⎪
   process ⎭
27 Spinous process
28 Costal fovea
29 Body
30 Head of rib
31 Costal cartilage

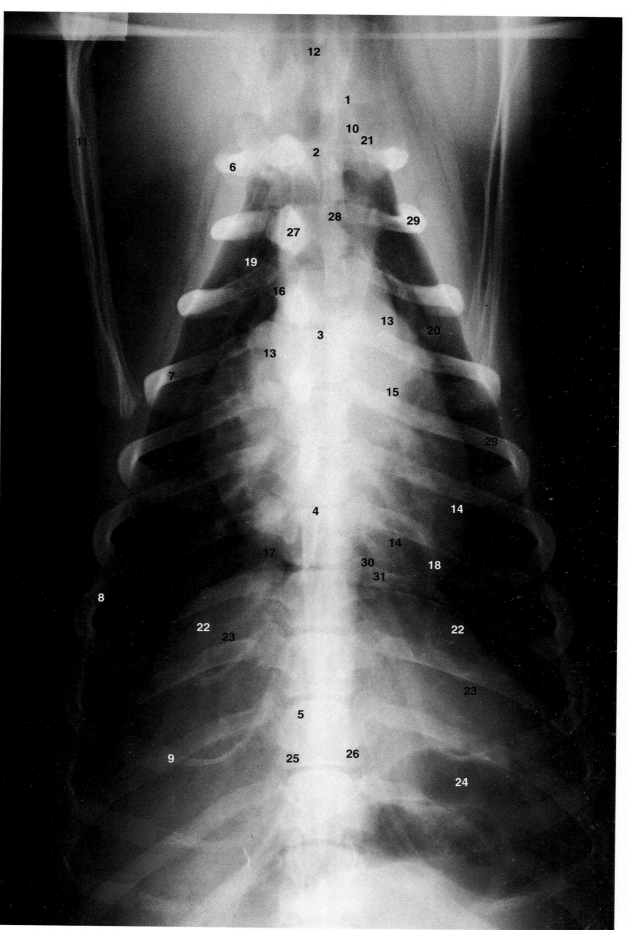

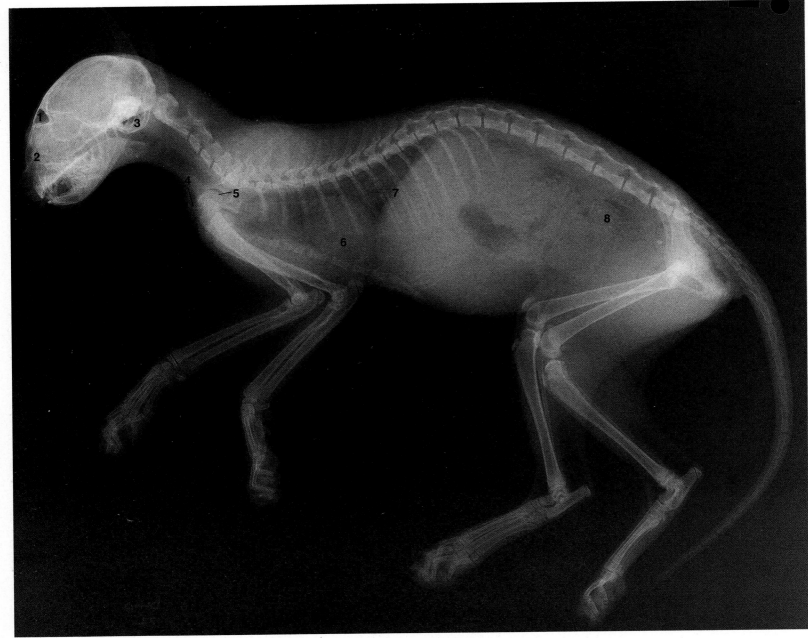

169 Lateral radiograph of a kitten, showing the skeletal elements and centres of ossification.

1	Frontal sinus	5	Suprahamate process on acromion of scapula
2	Maxilla	6	Heart
3	Tympanic bulla	7	Diaphragm
4	Clavicle	8	Descending colon

- The clavicle and the suprahamate process are not found in the dog.
- Note the foreshortened facial region of the skull.

170 **Dorsoventral radiograph of the head, neck and thorax of a cat.**

1	Canine teeth
2	Maxilla
3	Zygomatic arch
4	Mandible
5	Tympanic bulla
6	First cervical vertebra (atlas)
7	Second cervical vertebra (axis)
8	Manubrium sterni
9	First rib
10	Scapula
11	Suprahamate process
12	Clavicle
13	Humerus
14	Olecranon of ulna
15	Radius
16	Apex } of heart
17	Base
18	Diaphragm
19	First lumbar vertebra
20	Left } renal outline
21	Right

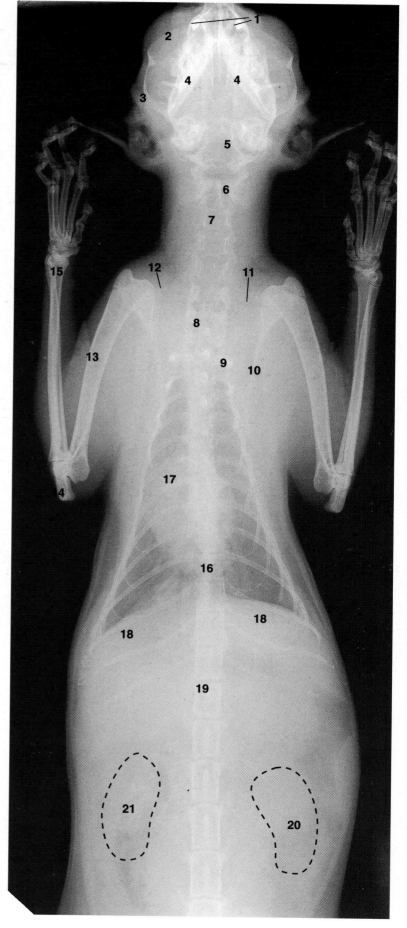

171   171 Cross section through the ventricles of a dog heart.

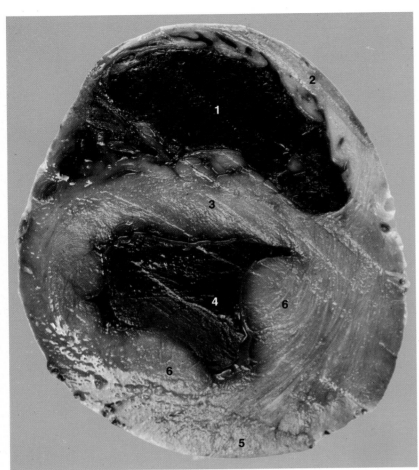

1	Lumen	} of right ventricle	4	Lumen	} of left ventricle
2	Free wall		5	Free wall	
3	Interventricular septum		6	Papillary muscles	

- This section through the ventricles gives an anatomical plane similar to that in a short-axis ultrasound scan. It is the preferred position for measuring ventricular dimensions with M-mode ultrasonography.

172

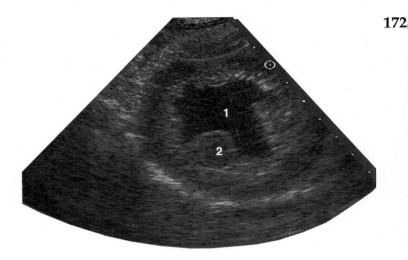

172 Ultrasound scan of a short-axis cross section through the left ventricle of the heart of a dog. The papillary muscles are seen at the periphery of the ventricle.

1	Left ventricle	2	Papillary muscle

173

173 Longitudinal section of the heart of a dog, showing the intracardiac structures seen on long-axis ultrasound scans.

1	Free wall	} of right ventricle
2	Lumen	
3	Interventricular septum	
4	Apex of heart	
5	Free wall of left ventricle	
6	Papillary muscle	
7	Chordae tendineae	
8	Coronary vessels	
9	Mitral (left atrioventricular) valve	
10	Left atrium	
11	Left auricle	
12	Outflow tract of left ventricle	
13	Aortic valve	
14	Aorta	
15	Pulmonary artery	
16	Base of heart	

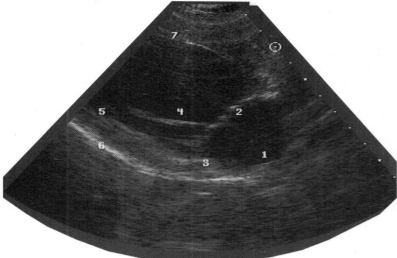

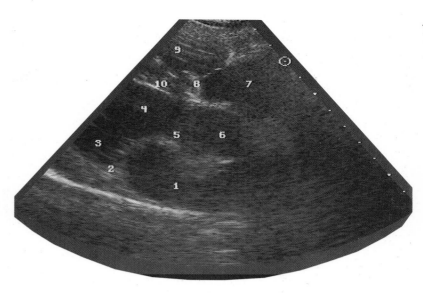

174 Ultrasound scan of the left ventricle of the heart of a dog, taken from the left thoracic wall. The plane of the scan is in the long axis and the encircled dot is cranial.

1	Left atrium	4	Chordae tendineae
2	Septal cusp of mitral (left	5	Papillary muscle in left ventricle
3	Parietal (free wall) cusp atrioventricular) valve	6	Free wall of left ventricle
		7	Interventricular septum

175 Ultrasound scan of the heart of a dog, taken from the right side of the thorax. The two atrioventricular valves and the aortic valve are displayed. The plane of the scan is in the long axis and the encircled dot is cranial.

1	Left atrium	7	Right atrium
2	Mitral (left atrioventricular) valve	8	Tricuspid (right atrioventricular) valve
3	Left ventricle	9	Right ventricle
4	Outflow tract of 3	10	Interventricular septum
5	Aortic valve		
6	Aorta		

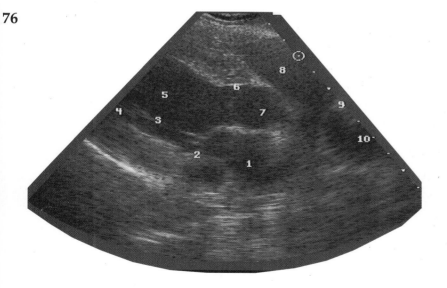

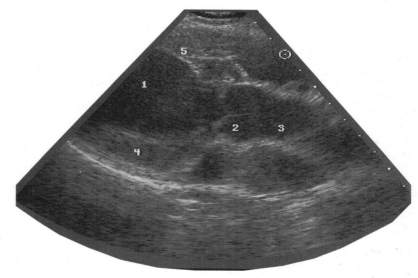

176 Ultrasound scan of the heart of a dog, taken from the left side of the thorax. The plane of the scan is in the long axis and the encircled dot is cranial.

1	Left atrium	7	Aorta
2	Mitral (left atrioventricular) valve	8	Right ventricle
3	Chordae tendineae	9	Tricuspid (right atrioventricular) valve
4	Papillary muscle	10	Right atrium
5	Outflow tract of left ventricle		
6	Aortic valve		

177 Ultrasound scan of the heart of a dog, taken from the left side of the thorax. The aortic valve is displayed. The plane of the scan is in the long axis and the encircled dot is cranial.

1	Outflow tract of left ventricle	4	Free wall of left ventricle
2	Aortic valve	5	Interventricular septum
3	Aorta		

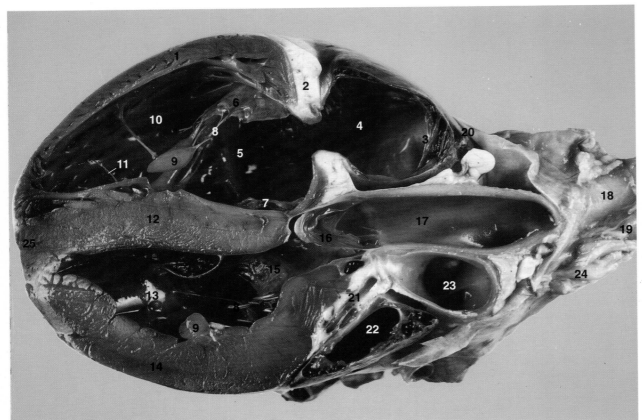

178 Longitudinal section through the heart of a dog, showing the right side and the outflow tract of the left ventricle.

1	Free wall of right ventricle
2	Coronary groove
3	Right auricle
4	Right atrium
5	Tricuspid (right atrioventricular) valve
6	Parietal (free wall) cusp
7	Septal cusp
8	Chordae tendineae
9	Papillary muscle
10	Lumen of right ventricle
11	Trabecula septomarginalis
12	Interventricular septum
13	Lumen ⎫
14	Free wall ⎬ of left ventricle
15	Outflow tract ⎭
16	Aortic valve
17	Aorta
18	Brachiocephalic trunk
19	Left subclavian artery
20	Pericardium (cut)
21	Coronary vessels
22	Left auricle
23	Pulmonary trunk
24	Base ⎫ of heart
25	Apex ⎭

179 Ultrasound scan of the right side of the heart of a dog, taken at the left thoracic wall. The apex of the heart is at the top of the scan.

1	Aortic valve
2	Left atrium
3	Right atrium
4	Tricuspid (right atrioventricular) valve
5	Right ventricle

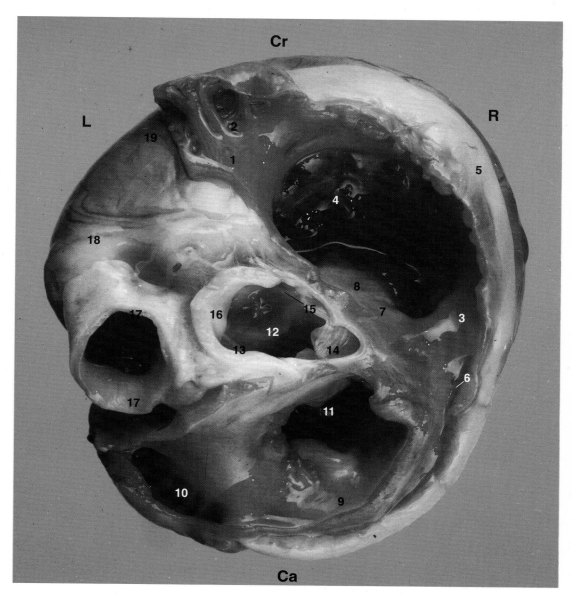

180 Dorsal aspect of the base of the heart of a dog, sectioned to reveal the valvular structures. The atria and auricles have been exposed, and the venae cavae and pulmonary veins removed. Cranial (Cr) and caudal (Ca) orientation are indicated.

1	Right auricle	11	Mitral (left atrioventricular) valve
2	Mm. pectinati	12	Right semilunar valvula
3	Right atrium	13	Left semilunar valvula } of aortic valve
4	Tricuspid (right atrioventricular) valve	14	Dorsal semilunar valvula
5	Coronary groove	15	Opening for right coronary artery from right sinus of aorta
6	Opening of coronary sinus	16	Aorta
7	Fossa ovalis	17	Pulmonary trunk
8	Intervenous tubercle	18	Conus arteriosus
9	Left atrium	19	Wall of right ventricle
10	Left auricle		

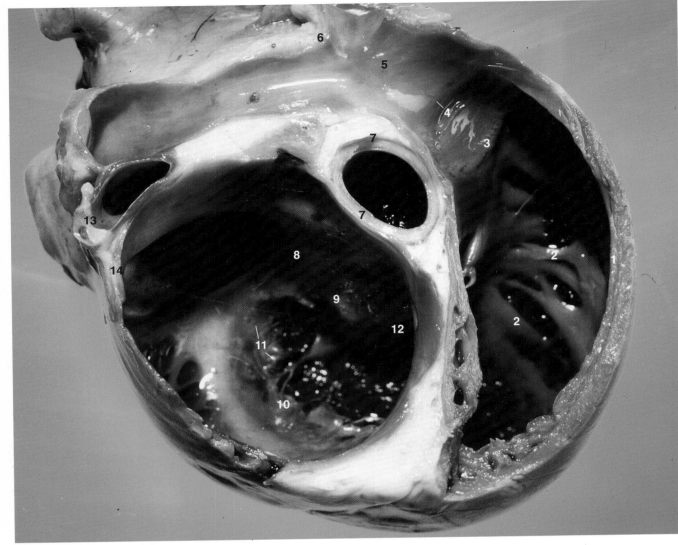

181 Oblique cross section through the heart of a dog, made at the level of the pulmonary valve to show the relationship with the aorta.

1	Free wall of right ventricle	9	Tricuspid (right atrioventricular) valve
2	Trabeculae carneae	10	Parietal (free wall) cusp
3	Outflow tract of right ventricle	11	Chordae tendineae
4	Pulmonary valve	12	Right ventricle
5	Pulmonary artery	13	Pulmonary vein
6	Bifurcation of 5	14	Right auricle
7	Aorta		
8	Right atrium		

- Note how the pulmonary trunk curls around the aorta.

- This is the scanning field used to interrogate the pulmonary valve in echocardiography.

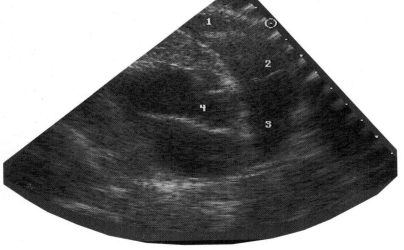

182 Ultrasound scan of the pulmonary valve of the heart of a dog, taken from the left thoracic wall. The pulmonary trunk can be seen curling around the aorta.

1	Outflow tract of right ventricle
2	Pulmonary valve
3	Pulmonary artery
4	Aortic valve

6 Abdomen and pelvic cavities

The bony framework of the abdominal and pelvic regions is first demonstrated before the layers of soft tissue structures have been exposed. The internal viscera of these regions are then comprehensively displayed using dissected and cross-sectional specimens, radiography and B-mode ultrasonography. Variations between the male and female organs including the external genitalia, are exhibited. Particular attention is paid to the topographical features of the abdomen and the pelvic cavities.

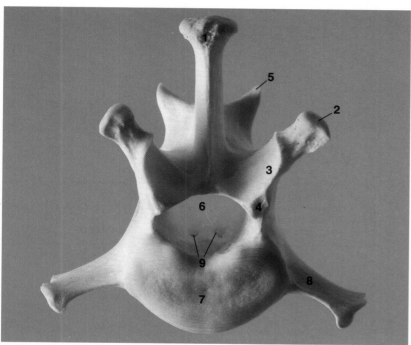

183 Cranial aspect of the first lumbar vertebra of a dog.

1	Spinous process	6	Vertebral foramen
2	Mamillary process	7	Body
3	Cranial articular surface	8	Transverse process
4	Cranial articular process	9	Dorsal foramina
5	Caudal articular process		

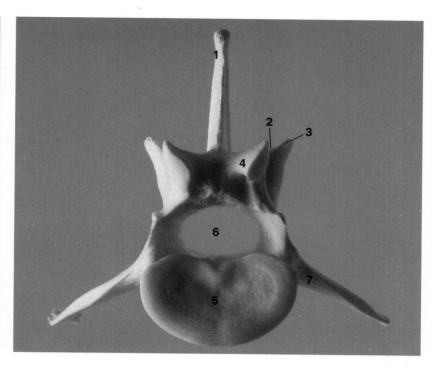

184 Caudal aspect of the fifth lumbar vertebra of a dog.

1	Spinous process	5	Body
2	Cranial articular process	6	Vertebral foramen
3	Mamillary process	7	Transverse process
4	Caudal articular process		

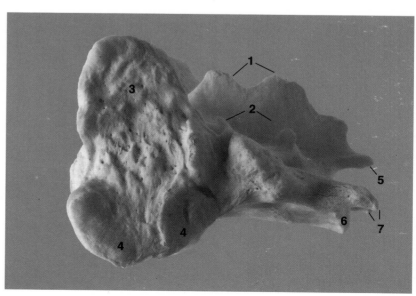

185 Lateral aspect of the sacrum of a dog.

1	Median sacral crest	5	Caudal articular process
2	Intermediate sacral crest	6	Body
3	Wing	7	Transverse process
4	Auricular surface		

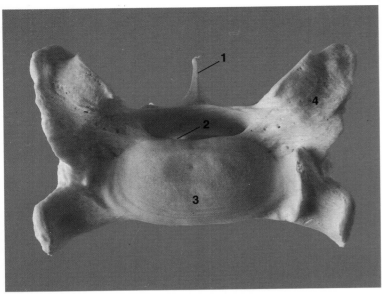

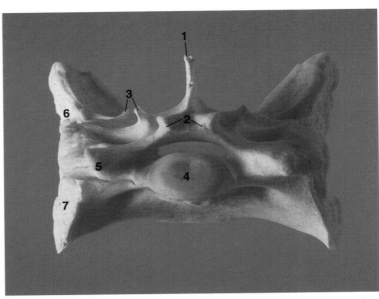

186 Cranial aspect of the sacrum of a dog.

187 Caudal aspect of the sacrum of a dog.

1	Spinous process of median sacral crest
2	Sacral canal
3	Base
4	Wing

1	Spinous process of median sacral crest	4	Body
2	Caudal articular process	5	Lateral sacral crest
3	Intermediate sacral crest	6	Wing
		7	Auricular surface

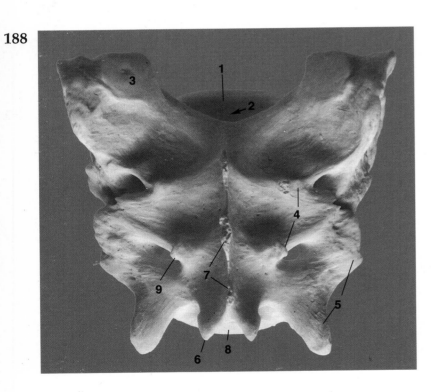

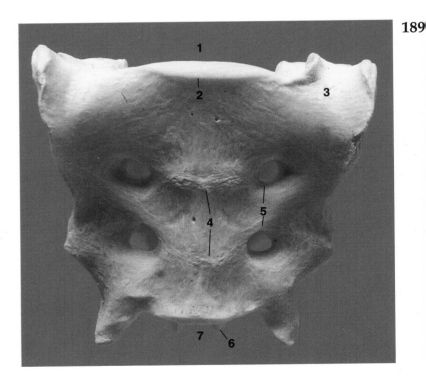

188 Dorsal aspect of the sacrum of a dog.

189 Ventral aspect of the sacrum of a dog.

1	Base	6	Caudal articular process
2	Sacral canal	7	Median sacral crest
3	Cranial articular surface	8	Apex
4	Intermediate sacral crest	9	Dorsal sacral foramina
5	Lateral sacral crest		

1	Base	5	Pelvic sacral foramina
2	Promontory	6	Caudal articular process
3	Wing	7	Apex
4	Transverse lines		

190 Dorsal aspect of the fifth caudal vertebra (A), ventral aspect of the fourth (B) and sixth (C) caudal vertebra, and dorsal aspect of the fourteenth caudal vertebra (D) of a dog.

1	Cranial articular process
2	Mamillary process
3	Neural arch
4	Caudal articular process
5	Transverse process
6	Haemal arch
7	Body
8	Cranial transverse process

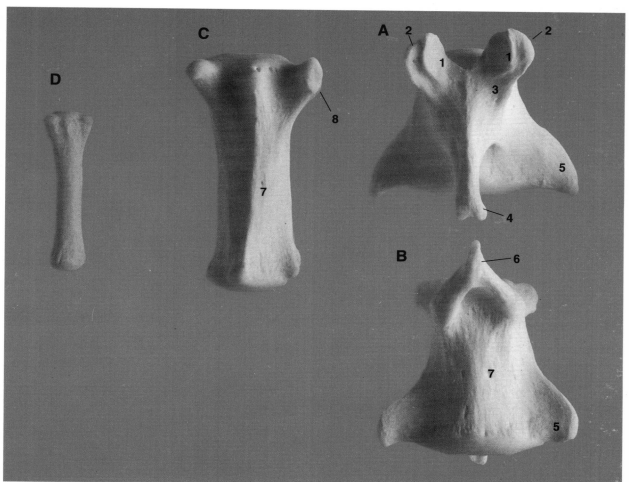

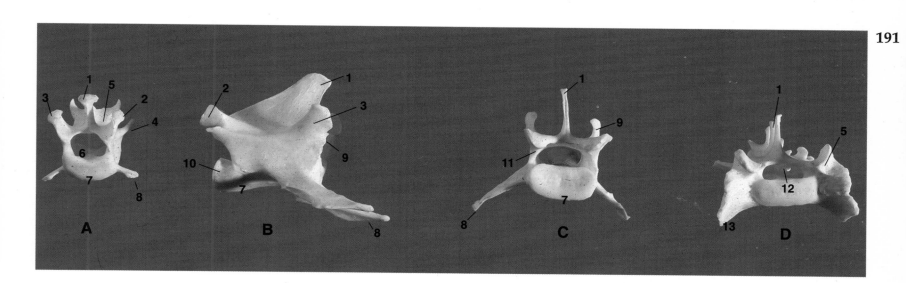

191 Cranial aspect of the first lumbar vertebra (A), lateral (right side) aspect of the fifth lumbar vertebra (B), caudal aspect of the seventh lumbar vertebra (C), and cranial aspect of the sacrum of a cat.

1	Spinous process	6	Vertebral foramen	11	Caudal articular surface
2	Caudal articular process	7	Body	12	Sacral canal
3	Mamillary process	8	Transverse process	13	Sacral wing
4	Accessory process	9	Cranial articular process		
5	Cranial articular surface	10	Caudal vertebral notch		

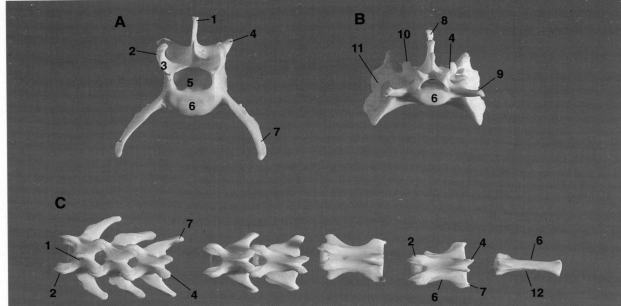

192 Cranial aspect of the seventh lumbar vertebra (A), caudal aspect of the sacrum (B), and dorsal aspect of the first, second, and third caudal vertebrae (C) of a cat.

1	Spinous process
2	Cranial articular process
3	Cranial articular surface
4	Caudal articular process
5	Vertebral foramen
6	Body
7	Transverse process
8	Spinous processes (median sacral crest)
9	Lateral crest
10	Intermediate sacral crest
11	Wing
12	Distal segment of caudal vertebra (dorsal)

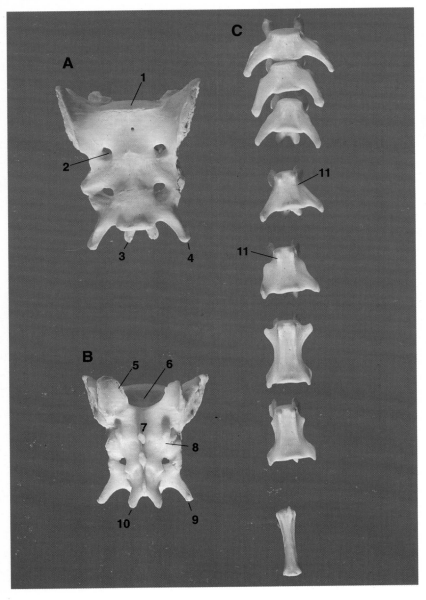

193 Ventral (A) and dorsal aspect (B) of the sacrum, and ventral aspect (C) of several caudal vertebrae of a cat.

1	Promontory	6	Sacral canal
2	Pelvic sacral foramina	7	Median sacral crest
3	Caudal articular surface	8	Intermediate sacral crest
4	Transverse process of lateral sacral crest	9	Lateral sacral crest
5	Cranial articular surface	10	Caudal articular process
		11	Haemal process

194 Lateral aspect of the articulated lumbar vertebrae of a dog.

1 First lumbar vertebra
2 Seventh lumbar vertebra
3 Body
4 Spinous process
5 Cranial articular process
6 Mamillary process
7 Caudal articular process
8 Transverse process
9 Accessory process
10 Intervertebral foramen

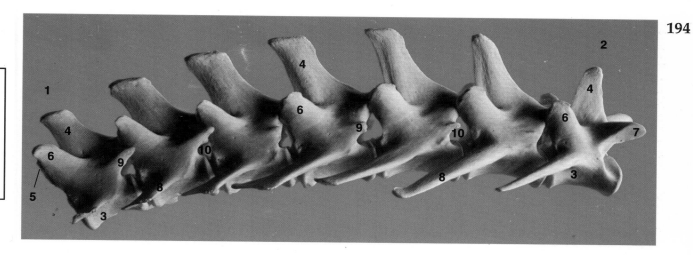

194

195 Dorsal aspect of the articulated lumbar vertebrae of a dog.

1 First lumbar vertebra
2 Seventh lumbar vertebra
3 Spinous process
4 Cranial articular process
5 Mamillary process
6 Caudal articular process
7 Transverse process
8 Accessory process

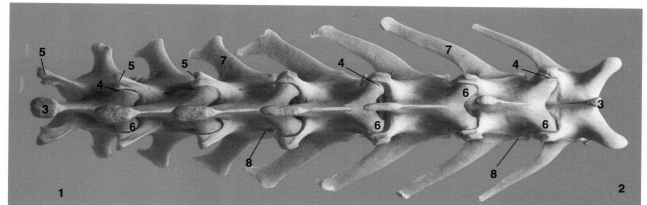

195

196 Radiograph of the lateral aspect of the lumbar region of the vertebral column of a dog.

1 Thirteenth thoracic vertebra
2 Thirteenth (floating) rib
3 First } lumbar vertebra
4 Seventh
5 Body of vertebra
6 Dorsal and ventral borders of vertebral foramen (vertebral canal)
7 Spinous process
8 Transverse process of lumbar vertebra
9 Intervertebral foramina
10 Cranial articular process
11 Caudal articular process
12 Accessory process
13 Body of sacrum
14 Wing of ilium

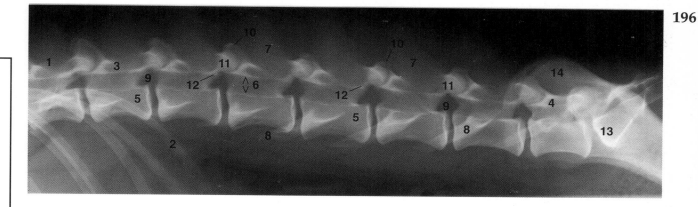

196

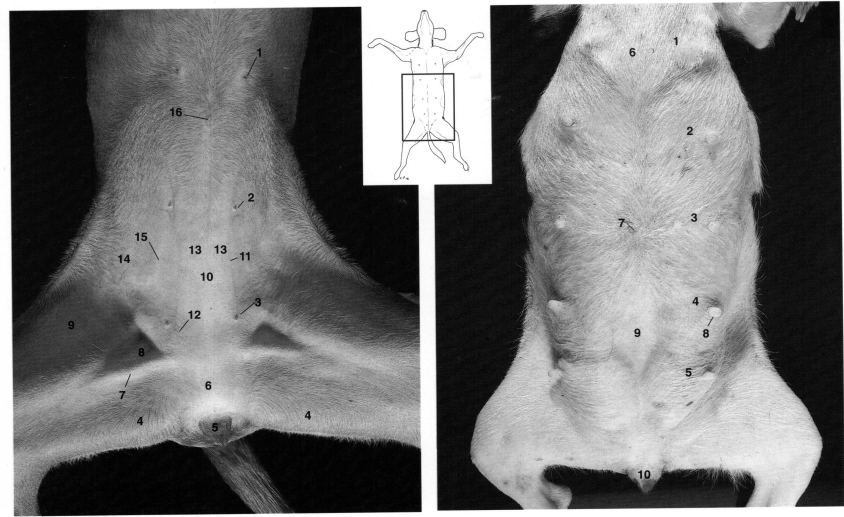

197 Ventral aspect of the intact abdominal wall and inguinal region of a nulliparous bitch.

198 Ventral aspect of the intact thoracic, abdominal and inguinal regions of a pregnant bitch.

1	Teat of cranial abdominal		10	Median raphe over linea alba
2	Teat of caudal abdominal	mammary gland	11	Caudal superficial epigastric artery and vein
3	Teat of inguinal abdominal		12	Level of superficial ring of inguinal canal
4	M. gracilis		13	M. rectus abdominis
5	Vulva		14	M. obliquus externus abdominis and m. obliquus internus abdominis
6	Symphysis pelvis			
7	M. pectineus		15	Lateral border of sheath of m. rectus abdominis
8	Femoral triangle			
9	M. sartorius		16	Umbilical scar

1	Cranial thoracic			sternum
2	Caudal thoracic	mammary gland	7	Umbilical scar
3	Cranial abdominal		8	Teat with orifices
4	Caudal abdominal		9	Median raphe overlying linea alba
5	Inguinal		10	Vulva
6	Level of xiphoid process of			

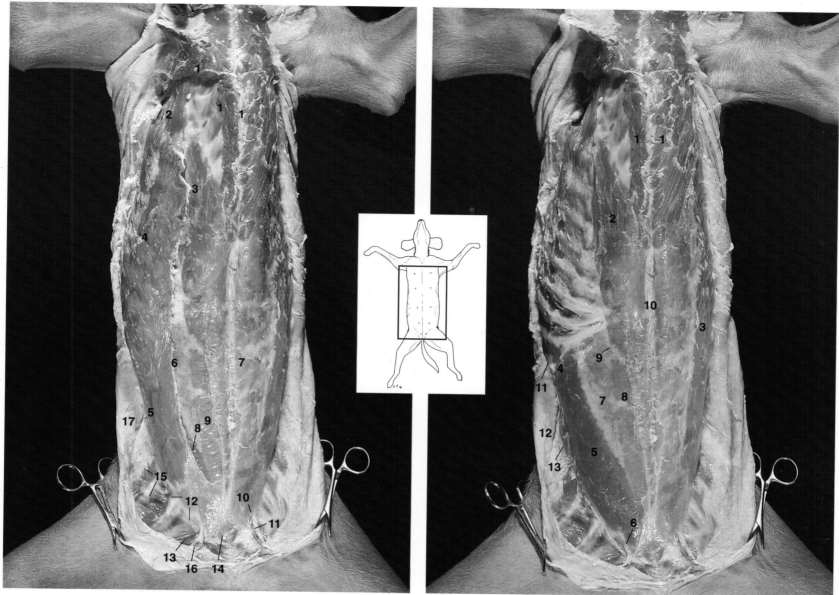

199 Ventral aspect of the thoracic and abdominal regions of a dog. The skin has been removed and the deep pectoral muscle reflected to reveal the muscles of the abdominal wall.

200 Ventral aspect of the thoracic and abdominal regions of a dog. The deep pectoral and external oblique abdominal muscles have been removed on the right side to reveal the internal oblique abdominal muscles.

1 M. pectoralis profundus	10 External inguinal ring
2 M. scalenus	11 Vaginal process with external
3 M. rectus abdominis	pudendal vessels
4 Pars costalis ⎫ of M. obliquus	12 Femoral triangle
5 Pars lumbalis ⎬ externus	13 M. pectineus
6 Aponeurosis ⎭ abdominis	14 Prepubic tendon
(cut edge)	15 M. sartorius
7 Sheath of M. rectus abdominis	16 Superficial inguinal lymph node
8 M. obliquus internus abdominis	17 Reflected skin
9 Contribution of 6 running in	
superficial sheath of M. rectus	
abdominis	

1 M. pectoralis profundus	internus abdominis in superficial
2 M. rectus abdominis	sheath of M. rectus abdominis
3 M. obliquus externus abdominis	9 Aponeurosis of M. obliquus
4 Pars costalis ⎫ of M.	internus abdominis running deep
5 Pars abdominis ⎬ obliquus	to M. rectus abdominis
6 Pars inguinalis (from ⎫ internus	10 Linea alba
inguinal ligament) ⎭ abdominis	11 Thirteenth (floating) rib
7 M. transversus abdominis seen	12 Reflected skin
through aponeurosis of M.	13 M. obliquus externus abdominis
obliquus internus abdominis	(cut edge)
8 Aponeurosis of M. obliquus	

- To gain surgical access to the abdominal cavity, incisions are made precisely in the midline ventrally, through the linea alba.

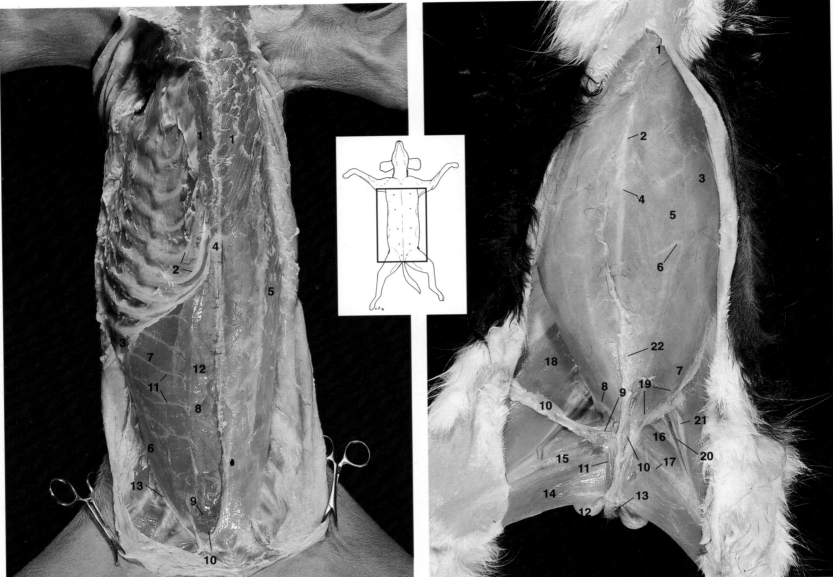

201 Ventral aspect of the thoracic and abdominal regions of a dog. The deep pectoral, external and internal oblique abdominal, and rectus muscles have been removed on the right side to reveal the deeper layers.

1	M. pectoralis profundus	10	M. rectus abdominis (cut edge)
2	Costal cartilages	11	Medial branches of ventral divisions of thoracic and lumbar nerves
3	Thirteenth rib (floating)		
4	Xiphoid process of sternum		
5	M. obliquus externus abdominis	12	Abdominal viscera seen through aponeurosis of 6 and 7, fascia transversalis and parietal peritoneum
6	Pars lumbalis		
7	Pars costalis		
8	Aponeurosis lying deep to 10 (resected)	of M. transversus abdominis	
		13	M. obliquus internus abdominis (cut edge)
9	Aponeurosis lying superficial to 10		

202 Ventral aspect of the superficial abdominal muscles of a male cat.

1	M. pectoralis profundus	11	Spermatic cord
2	Linea alba	12	Testis
3	M. obliquus externus abdominis	13	Prepuce
4	Umbilical scar	14	M. gracilis
5	Superficial sheath	of M. rectus abdominis	15	M. adductor
6	Tendinous inscriptions		16	M. pectineus
7	M. obliquus internus abdominis seen through aponeurotic sheet of M. obliquus externus abdominus	17	Branch of obturator nerve
		18	M. sartorius
8	External inguinal ring	19	Femoral triangle
9	External pudendal artery and vein	20	Femoral artery and vein
10	Chain of superficial inguinal lymph nodes	21	Saphenous nerve (branch of femoral nerve)
		22	Subcutaneous fat

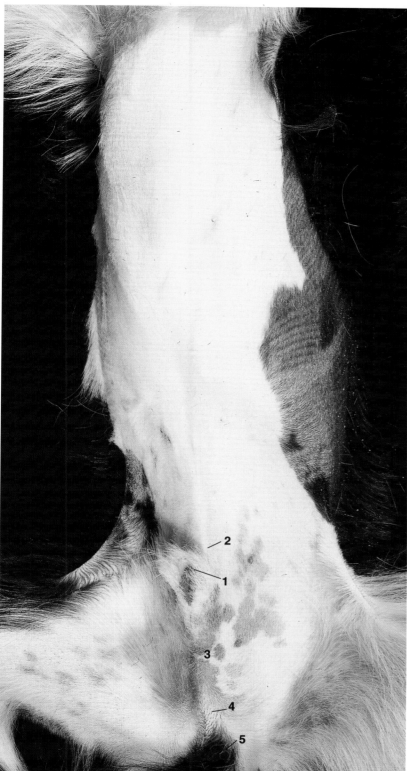

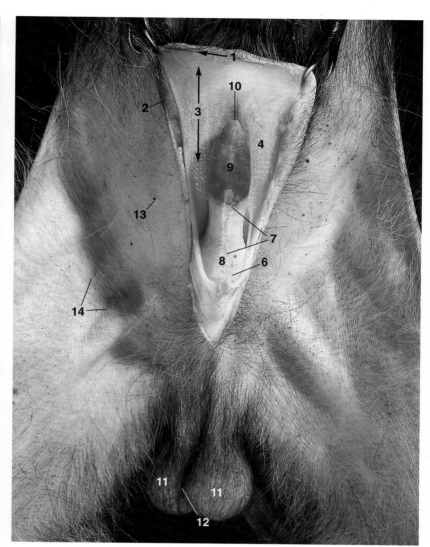

204 Ventral aspect of the inguinal region of a male dog. The prepuce has been opened ventrally to expose the preputial cavity and the glans penis.

1	Preputial orifice (opened ventrally)	9	Pars longa glandis
2	Outer surface ⎱ of prepuce	10	External urethral orifice
3	External lamina ⎰	11	Scrotal sacs
4	Lymph nodules	12	Median raphe
5	M. preputialis	13	Teat of undeveloped inguinal mammary gland
6	Fornix		
7	Internal lamina of prepuce	14	Femoral triangle
8	Bulbus glandis		

203 Ventral aspect of the prepuce of a male dog.

1	Preputial orifice
2	Median fold
3	Glans penis within prepuce
4	Caudal extremity of os penis
5	Scrotum

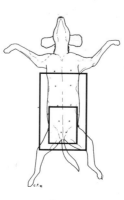

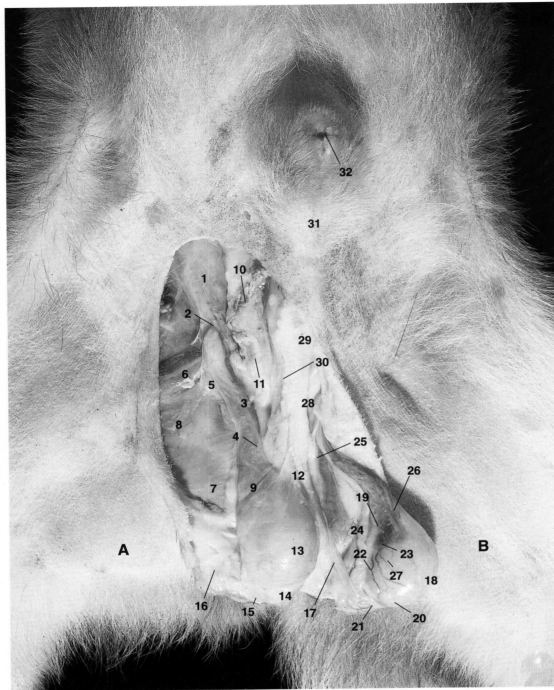

Ventral aspect of the inguinal region of a male dog. The scrotal wall has been sectioned on the right side (A) to reveal the testis within the parietal layer of the vaginal tunic. On the left side (B) the parietal layer has been resected to expose the visceral layer of the vaginal tunic covering the testis.

1	M. obliquus externus abdominis
2	Superficial inguinal ring
3	Spermatic cord
4	Vaginal process
5	External abdominal fascia
6	M. pectineus
7	M. gracilis
8	M. adductor
9	M. cremaster within spermatic cord
10	External pudendal artery and vein
11	Superficial inguinal lymph node
12	Spermatic fascia
13	Testis within parietal layer of vaginal tunic
14	Tail of epididymis
15	Scrotal ligament
16	Scrotal wall
17	Median scrotal septum
18	Testis covered in visceral layer of vaginal tunic
19	Ductus deferens
20	Proper ligament of testis
21	Ligament of tail of epididymis
22	Artery and vein of ductus deferens
23	Mesoductus deferens
24	M. cremaster
25	Parietal layer of vaginal tunic
26	Pampiniform plexus of veins
27	Testicular veins
28	Body
29	Bulbus glandis } of penis
30	Dorsal artery and vein
31	Prepuce
32	Preputial orifice

- The exposure of the testis on the right side (A) represents the field seen in the technique of closed castration, and on the left side (B), that seen in open castration.

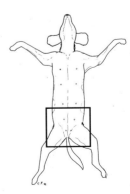

206 Caudal aspect of the perineum of male cat.

1 M. sacrocaudalis ventralis lateralis
2 M. rectococcygeus
3 M. coccygeus
4 M. levator ani
5 M. sphincter ani externus
6 Anus
7 Position of anal sac
8 M. retractor penis overlying M. bulbospongiosum
9 Body of penis
10 M. ischiocavernosus
11 Ischiatic tuberosity
12 Glans penis
13 External urethral orifice
14 Prepuce (opened)
15 Testis covered by parietal layer of vaginal tunic
16 Spermatic cord
17 Sacrotuberous ligament (vestigial)
18 M. obturator internus
19 M. gluteus superficialis
20 M. abductor cruris cranialis (M. coccygeofemoralis)
21 M. biceps femoris
22 M. semitendinosus
23 M. semimembranosus

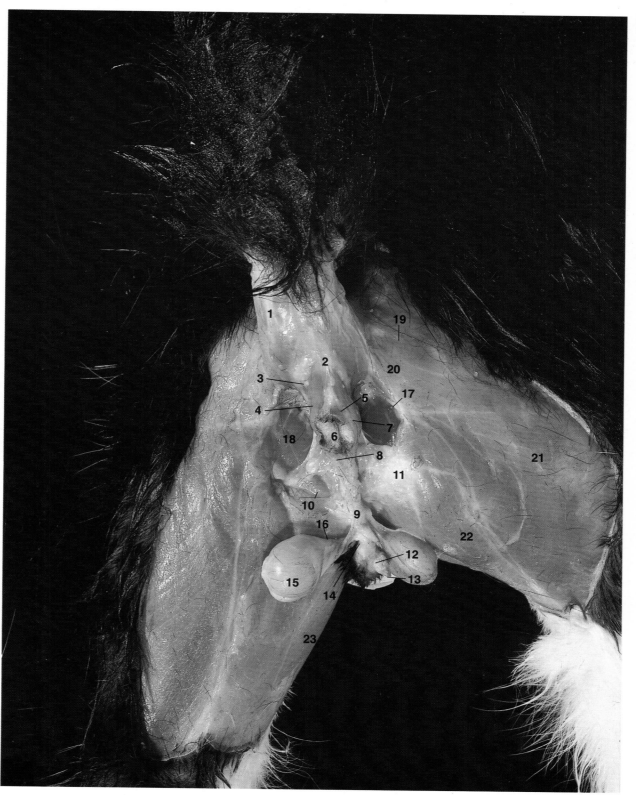

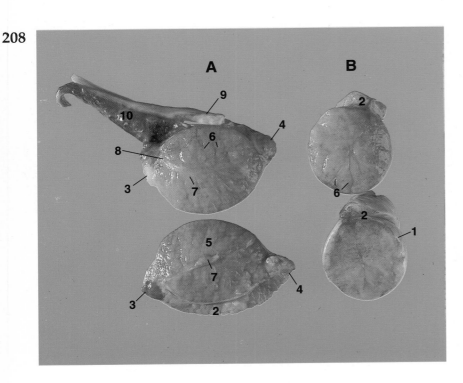

207 Lateral (A) and medial (B) aspect of the testes of a dog, after removal from the scrotal sacs and severance of the spermatic cords.

1	Pampiniform plexus of veins
2	Ductus deferens
3	Testis covered in visceral vaginal tunic
4	Head (extremitas capitata) } of testis
5	Tail (extremitas caudata) } of testis
6	Head
7	Body } of epididymis
8	Sinus } of epididymis
9	Tail
10	Parietal layer of vaginal tunic
11	M. cremaster
12	Mesofuniculus
13	External spermatic fascia
14	Proper ligament of testis
15	Ligament of tail of epididymis

208 Longitudinal (A) and transverse (B) sections of the testis of a dog.

1	Tunica albuginea (covered in visceral layer of vaginal tunic)	6	Connective tissue septa
2	Body	7	Mediastinum testis
3	Head } of epididymis	8	Rete testis
4	Tail } of epididymis	9	Ductus deferens
5	Parenchyma testis	10	Pampiniform plexus of veins

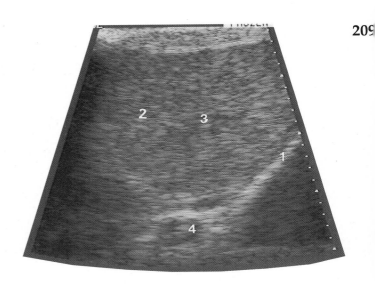

209 Cross-sectional ultrasound scan of the testis of a dog.

1	Tunica albuginea
2	Parenchyma testis
3	Mediastinum
4	Epididymis

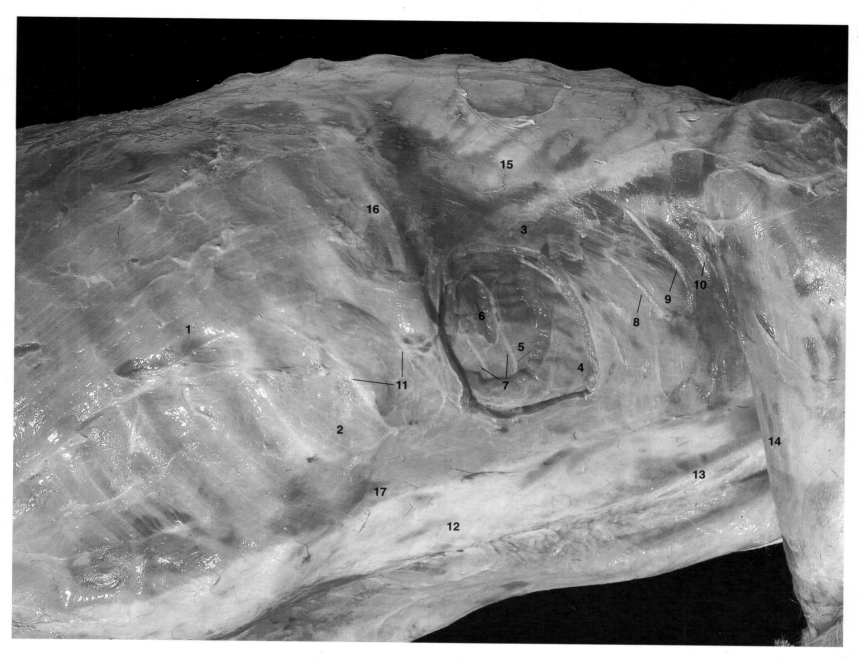

210 Lateral aspect of the left lateral abdominal region of a dog. The skin has been reflected to reveal the muscles of the region, and the abdominal muscle layers have been serially sectioned.

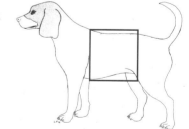

1	M. latissimus dorsi
2	Pars costalis ⎫ of M. obliquus
3	Pars lumbalis ⎭ externus abdominis
4	M. obliquus internus abdominis
5	M. transversus
6	Fascia transversalis
7	Ventral divisions of last thoracic and first lumbar nerves
8	Caudal iliohypogastric nerve

(ventral branch of second lumbar nerve)
9 Ilioinguinal nerve (ventral branch of third lumbar nerve)
10 Lateral cutaneous femoral nerve (ventral branch of fourth lumbar nerve)
11 Distal lateral cutaneous branches of intercostal nerves

12 Aponeurosis of M. obliquus externus abdominis
13 M. rectus abdominis (deep to 12)
14 M. sartorius
15 Thoracolumbar fascia
16 Thirteenth (floating) rib
17 Costal arch of costal cartilages

• This dissection of the lateral abdominal wall represents the muscle layers encountered when performing a surgical lateral flank abdominal incision.

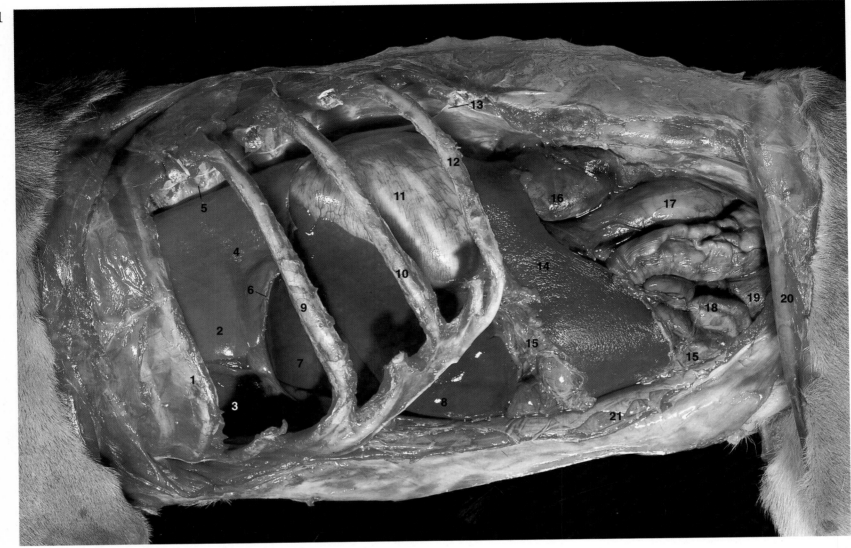

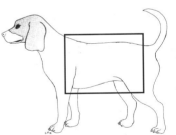

211 Left lateral aspect of the thoracic and abdominal regions of the dog. The thoracic and abdominal lateral walls have been removed, together with the diaphragm, to reveal the topography of the regions.

1	Sixth rib	12	Twelfth rib
2	Caudal part of cranial lobe of left lung	13	Thirteenth (floating) rib
3	Heart	14	Spleen
4	Caudal lobe of left lung	15	Greater omentum
5	Sympathetic trunk	16	Left kidney
6	Diaphragm (cut)	17	Descending colon
7	Left medial lobe } of liver	18	Jejunum
8	Left lateral lobe	19	Urinary bladder
9	Eighth rib	20	M. sartorius
10	Tenth rib	21	M. rectus abdominis
11	Stomach		

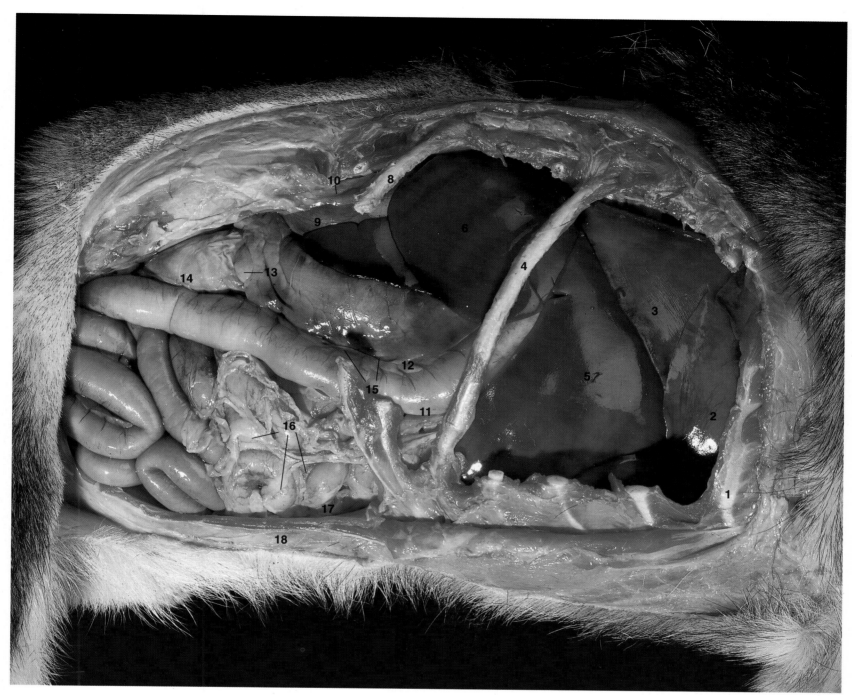

212 Lateral aspect of the thoracic and abdominal regions of a dog. The thoracic and abdominal lateral walls have been removed, together with the diaphragm, to reveal the topography of the region.

1	Eighth rib	10	Thirteenth (floating) rib
2	Middle lobe ⎫ of right lung	11	Descending duodenum
3	Caudal lobe ⎭	12	Pancreas
4	Tenth rib	13	Caecum
5	Right medial lobe ⎫ of liver	14	Descending colon
6	Right lateral lobe ⎬ (against diaphragm)	15	Mesoduodenum
7	Caudate lobe ⎭	16	Greater omentum
8	Twelfth rib	17	Jejunum
9	Right kidney	18	M. rectus abdominis

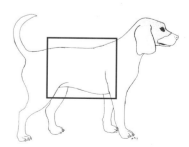

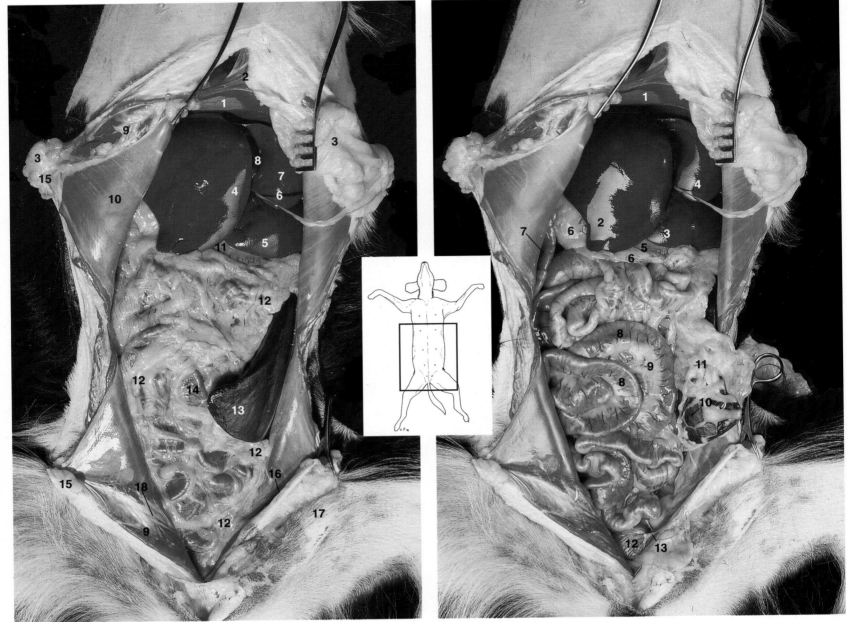

213 Ventral aspect of the opened abdomen of a male dog. The abdominal wall has been sectioned longitudinally in the midline ventrally, along the linea alba, and in a transverse direction at the level of the umbilicus. The greater omentum is seen *in situ*.

214 Ventral aspect of the opened abdomen of a male dog. The greater omentum has been reflected cranially to reveal the coils of the intestinal tract.

1	Diaphragm	10	M. transversus abdominis
2	Xiphoid process of sternum	11	Greater curvature of stomach
3	Falciform ligament	12	Greater omentum
4	Right medial lobe ⎫	13	Spleen
5	Left lateral lobe ⎬ of liver	14	Jejunum through 12
6	Quadrate lobe ⎮	15	Umbilicus
7	Left medial lobe ⎭	16	Linea alba
8	Gall bladder	17	Prepuce (reflected)
9	Deep aspect of M. rectus abdominis	18	Caudal deep epigastric artery and vein

1	Diaphragm	8	Jejunum
2	Right medial lobe ⎫	9	Great mesentery
3	Left lateral lobe ⎬ of liver	10	Spleen
4	Left medial lobe ⎭	11	Gastrosplenic ligament
5	Greater curvature of stomach	12	Urinary bladder
6	Greater omentum (reflected)	13	Median ligament of the bladder
7	Duodenum		

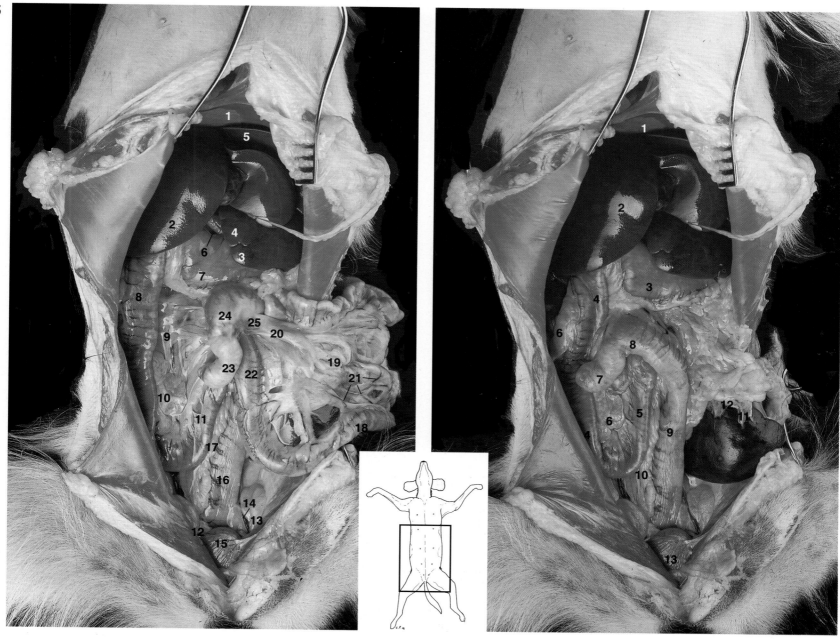

215 Ventral aspect of the open abdomen of a male dog. The greater omentum has been resected from the greater curvature of the stomach, and the coils of the jejunum have been displaced to reveal the ileocolic junction.

216 Ventral aspect of the opened abdomen of a male dog. The intestine has been removed from the level of the ascending duodenum to the ascending colon, and the spleen has been displaced to the left.

1	Diaphragm	14	Testicular vein
2	Right medial lobe	15	Urinary bladder
3	Left lateral lobe ⎫ of liver	16	Descending colon
4	Quadrate lobe	17	Mesocolon
5	Left medial lobe ⎭	18	Jejunum
6	Lesser curvature ⎫ of stomach	19	Great mesentery
7	Greater curvature ⎭	20	Mesenteric lymph nodes under fat
8	Descending duodenum	21	Branches of cranial mesenteric arteries and veins
9	Mesoduodenum	22	Ileum
10	Right lobe of pancreas	23	Caecum
11	Ascending duodenum	24	Ascending colon
12	Internal inguinal opening	25	Root of mesentery
13	Vaginal process		

1	Diaphragm	8	Transverse colon
2	Liver	9	Descending colon
3	Parietal surface of stomach	10	Mesocolon
4	Descending duodenum	11	Hilus of spleen
5	Ascending duodenum	12	Gastrosplenic ligament
6	Pancreas in mesoduodenum	13	Urinary bladder
7	Ascending colon		

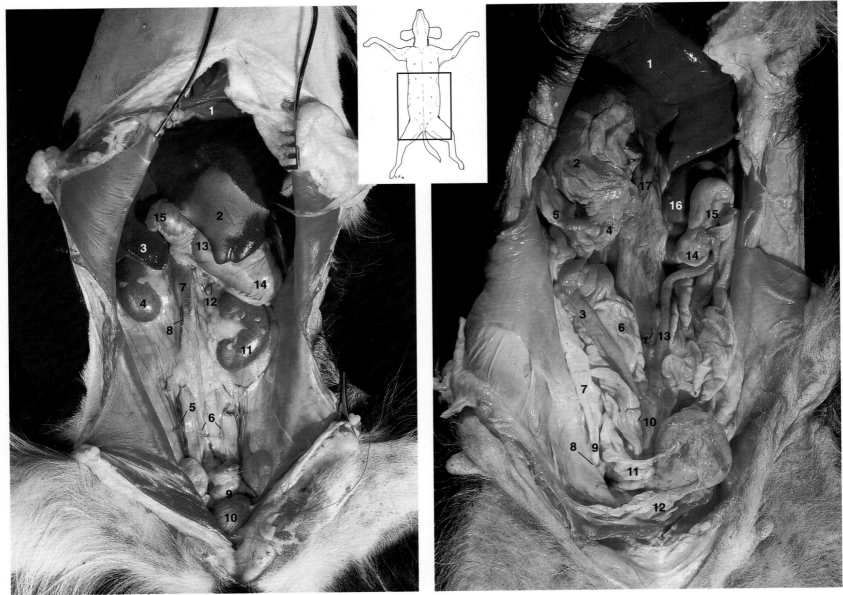

217 Ventral aspect of the opened abdomen of a male dog. The entire intestinal tract has been removed from the level of the pylorus to the descending colon at the pelvic inlet.

1	Diaphragm	8	Testicular vein
2	Right medial lobe	9	Descending colon (transected)
3	Caudate process } of liver	10	Urinary bladder
	of caudate lobe	11	Left kidney
4	Right kidney	12	Adrenal gland
5	Testicular artery and vein	13	Pylorus } of stomach
6	Ureters	14	Fundus
7	Caudal vena cava	15	Duodenum (transected)

218 Ventral aspect of the opened abdomen of a bitch. The gastrointestinal tract has been removed to reveal the urogenital tract *in situ*.

1	Liver	10	Uterine body
2	Caudal pole of right kidney	11	Lateral ligament } of bladder
3	Right uterine horn	12	Median ligament
4	Right ovary within ovarian bursa	13	Left uterine horn
5	Suspensory ligament	14	Left ovary within ovarian bursa
6	Mesometrium	15	Mesovarium with ovarian blood vessels
7	Round ligament of uterus	16	Left kidney
8	Internal opening of inguinal canal	17	Caudal vena cava
9	Vaginal process		

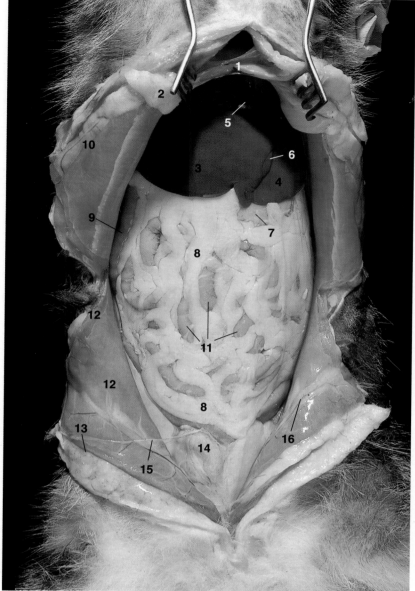

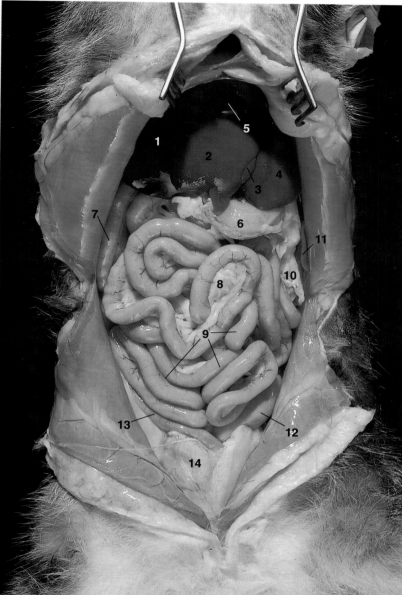

219 Ventral aspect of the opened abdomen of a cat. The muscles of the abdominal wall have been reflected to reveal the abdominal contents covered by the greater omentum.

1	Xiphoid process of sternum	11	Jejunum
2	Fat-laden falciform ligament	12	M. rectus abdominis
3	Right medial lobe ⎫ of liver	13	M. obliquus externus, internus M.
4	Left lateral lobe ⎭		obliquus abdominis and M.
5	Gall bladder		transversus abdominis
6	Quadrate lobe of liver	14	Urinary bladder
7	Stomach	15	Median ligament of bladder
8	Greater omentum	16	Deep caudal epigastric vessels
9	Descending duodenum		
10	Parietal peritoneum overlying deep rectal sheath		

220 Ventral aspect of the opened abdomen of a cat. The greater omentum has been resected at its attachment to the greater curvature of the stomach.

1	Right lateral lobe ⎫	8	Great mesentery
2	Right medial lobe ⎬ of liver	9	Jejunum
3	Quadrate lobe ⎮	10	Gastrosplenic ligament
4	Left lateral lobe ⎭	11	Spleen
5	Gall bladder	12	Descending colon
6	Greater curvature of stomach	13	Right uterine horn
7	Descending duodenum	14	Urinary bladder

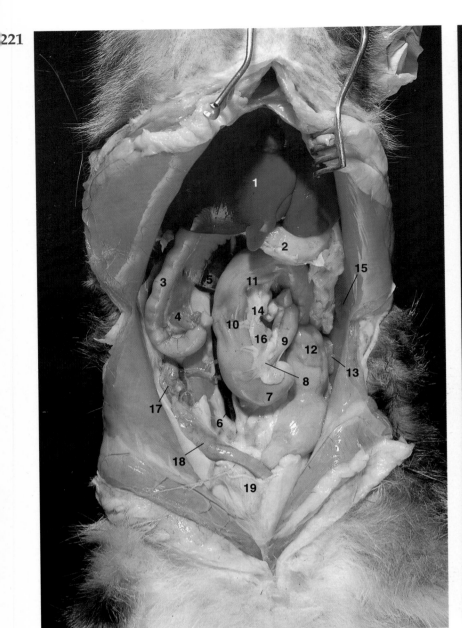

221 Ventral aspect of the opened abdomen of a female cat. The small intestine has been resected at the level of the descending duodenum and the terminal portion of the ileum.

222 Ventral aspect of the opened abdomen of a female cat. The intestinal tract has been removed to reveal the urogenital tract *in situ.*

1	Liver	10	Ascending colon
2	Stomach	11	Transverse colon
3	Duodenum	12	Descending colon
4	Right lobe of pancreas (in mesoduodenum)	13	Left ovary
		14	Root of mesentery
5	Caudate lobe of liver	15	Spleen
6	Caudal vena cava	16	Mesenteric lymph nodes
7	Caecum	17	Right ovary
8	Ileocolic junction	18	Right uterine horn
9	Ileum	19	Urinary bladder

1	Liver	16	Proper ligament of ovary
2	Caudate lobe of 1	17	Mesovarium
3	Right kidney	18	Ovarian artery and vein
4	Caudal vena cava	19	Uterine tube
5	Duodenum (cut)	20	Round ligament running to internal inguinal ring
6	Stomach	21	Uterine branch of 18
7	Spleen	22	Right uterine horn
8	Left kidney	23	M. psoas
9	Renal vein	24	Descending colon (cut)
10	Ovarian vessel	25	Urinary bladder
11	Aorta	26	Lateral aspect of left ovary
12	Ureter	27	Uterine tube
13	Suspensory ligament ⎱ of right	28	Left uterine horn
14	Medial aspect ⎰ ovary	29	Mesometrium
15	Entrance to ovarian bursa		

223 Dorsal aspect of the kidney of a dog.

1	Convex lateral border
2	Cranial pole
3	Medial border
4	Hilus
5	Renal artery
6	Renal vein
7	Ureter
8	Caudal pole

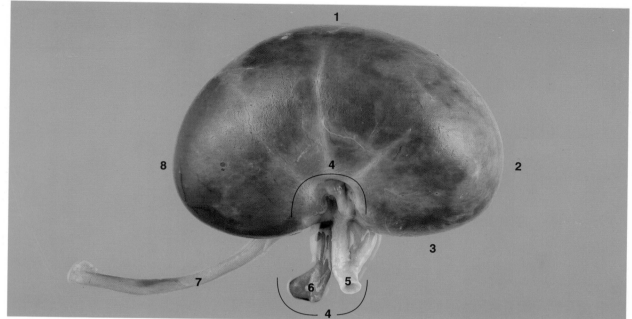

224 Dorsal aspect of a midfrontal section (A), and cross section (B) of the kidney of a dog.

1	Cortex with medullary rays
2	Medulla
3	Crest
4	Renal pelvis
5	Interlobar arteries and veins breaking up to form arcuate vessels
6	Sinus
7	Fat
8	Hilus
9	Renal artery
10	Ureter
11	Renal capsule

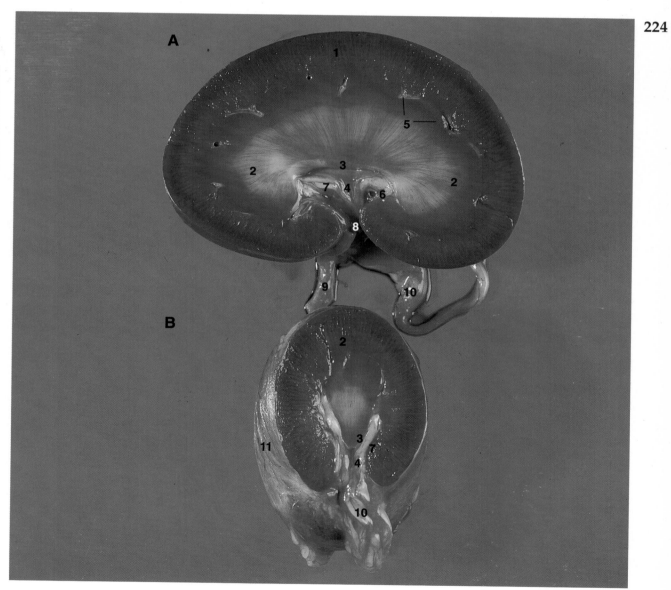

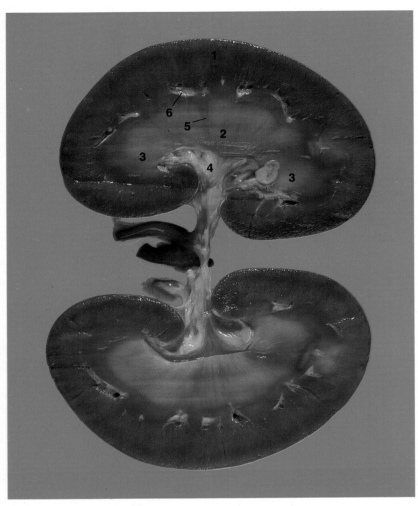

225 Frontal section in the dorsal plane, of the kidney of a dog.

1	Cortex
2	Pyramid
3	Medulla
4	Fat (in sinus)
5	Interlobar vessels
6	Arcuate vessels

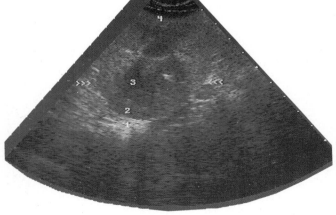

226 Transverse ultrasound scan of the kidney of a dog, illustrating the contrast between the echogenicity of the cortex and that of the medulla.

1	Kidney	3	Medulla
2	Cortex	4	Abdominal wall

- This scan is in a plane similar to that in the gross anatomical sectioned kidney.

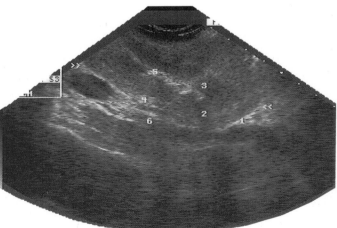

227 Ultrasound scan of the kidney of a dog, made in the dorsal plane, illustrating the contrast between the echogenicity of the cortex and that of the medulla. The renal pelvis produces strong echoes and appears white at the centre of the kidney outline.

1	Kidney	4	Hilus
2	Cortex	5	Renal pelvis
3	Medulla	6	Renal vessels

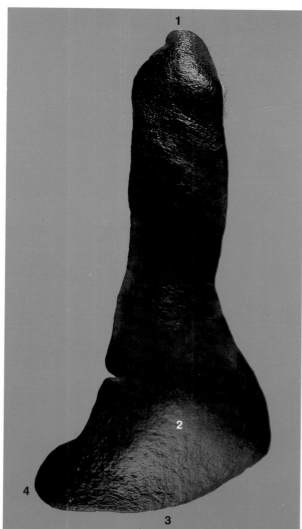

228 Parietal surface of the spleen of a dog.

1	Dorsal extremity
2	Parietal surface
3	Ventral extremity
4	Cranially directed tip

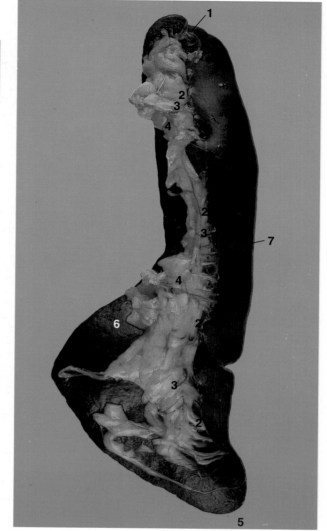

229 Visceral surface of the spleen of a dog.

1	Dorsal extremity
2	Hilus
3	Attachment of gastrosplenic ligament
4	Branches of splenic artery and vein
5	Ventral extremity
6	Intestinal surface
7	Gastric surface

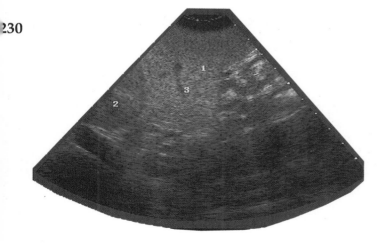

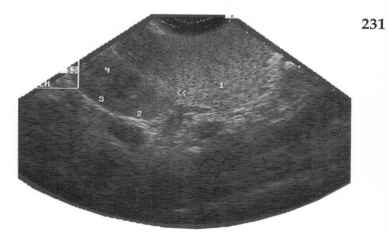

230 Ultrasound scan of the spleen of a dog, showing the splenic vessels running through the splenic tissue.

1	Spleen
2	Pole of kidney
3	Splenic vessels

231 Ultrasound scan of the kidney and spleen of a dog, illustrating the contrast in echogenicity between these organs. On the left, the spleen can be seen to abutt onto the kidney.

1	Spleen
2	Kidney
3	Renal cortex
4	Renal medulla

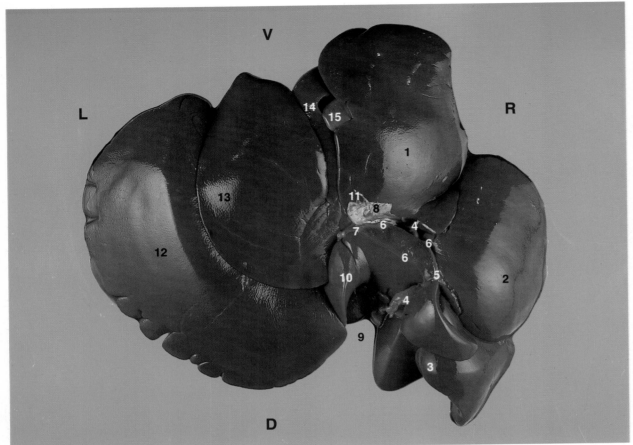

232 Diaphragmatic surface of the liver of a dog. Orientation ventrally (V), dorsally (D), left (L) and right (R) is indicated.

1	Right medial lobe
2	Right lateral lobe
3	Caudate lobe
4	Caudal vena cava
5	Right triangular ligament
6	Coronary ligament
7	Left triangular ligament
8	Fragment of diaphragm
9	Oesophageal notch
10	Papillary process of caudate lobe
11	Falciform ligament
12	Left lateral lobe
13	Left medial lobe
14	Quadrate lobe
15	Gall bladder

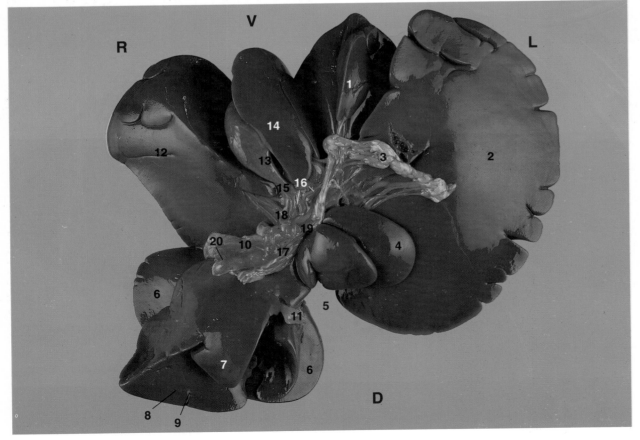

233 Visceral surface of the liver of a dog. Orientation ventrally (V), dorsally (D), left (L) and right (R) is indicated.

1	Left medial lobe
2	Left lateral lobe
3	Lesser omentum (hepatogastric ligament)
4	Papillary process of caudate lobe
5	Oesophageal notch
6	Right lateral lobe
7	Caudate process of caudate lobe
8	Renal fossa
9	Hepatorenal ligament
10	Lesser omentum (hepatoduodenal ligament)
11	Caudal vena cava
12	Right medial lobe
13	Gall bladder
14	Quadrate lobe
15	Cystic duct
16	Hepatic ducts
17	Bile duct
18	Portal vein
19	Hepatic artery
20	Gastroduodenal artery

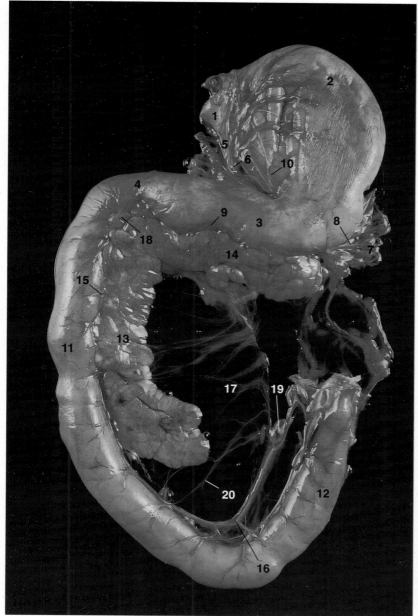

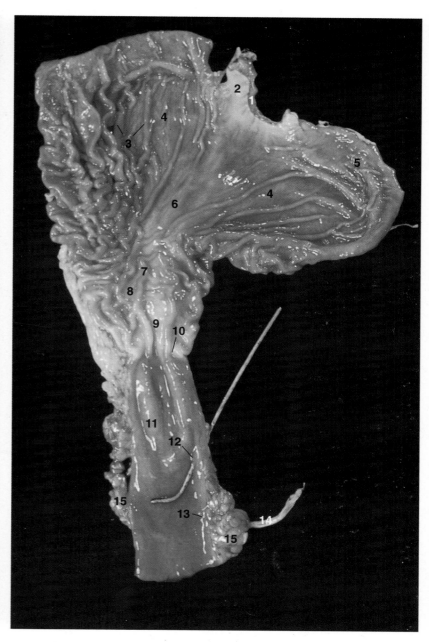

234 Ventral aspect of the stomach, duodenum and pancreas of a dog.

1	Cardia	13	Right lobe ⎫ of pancreas
2	Fundus	14	Left lobe ⎭
3	Pyloric antrum	15	Cranial pancreaticoduodenal
4	Pylorus		artery (from coeliac artery)
5	Lesser omentum	16	Caudal pancreaticoduodenal
6	Left gastric artery		artery (from cranial mesenteric
7	Greater omentum		artery)
8	Left gastroepiploic artery	17	Mesoduodenum
9	Right gastroepiploic artery	18	Duodenal lymph node
10	Lymphatic vessels	19	Mesenteric lymph node
11	Descending duodenum	20	Gastroduodenal branches of
12	Ascending duodenum		autonomic nerve fibres

235 Opened stomach of a dog. The organ has been cut along its greater curvature to reveal the mucosal lining. The probe occupies the point of entry of the major duodenal papilla.

1	Cardia	9	Pyloric canal
2	Region of cardiac glands	10	Pylorus
3	Gastric folds	11	Duodenum
4	Region of gastric glands (proper)	12	Major duodenal papilla (with probe)
5	Fundus	13	Minor duodenal papilla
6	Body	14	Pancreatic duct
7	Region of pyloric glands	15	Pancreatic tissue
8	Pyloric antrum		

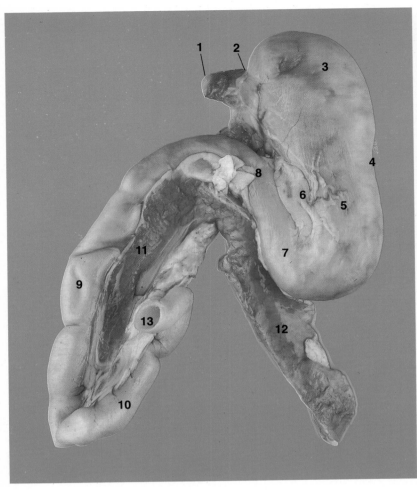

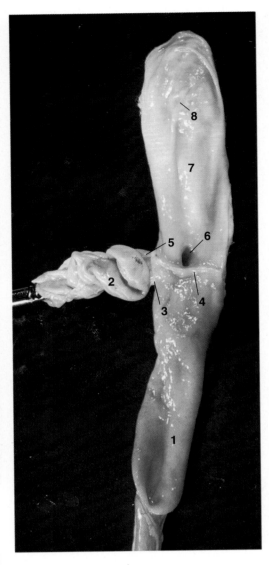

236 Stomach, duodenum and pancreas of a cat.

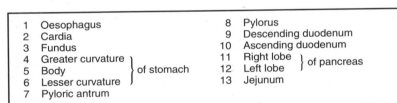

1	Oesophagus	8	Pylorus	
2	Cardia	9	Descending duodenum	
3	Fundus	10	Ascending duodenum	
4	Greater curvature	11	Right lobe	of pancreas
5	Body	12	Left lobe	
6	Lesser curvature	13	Jejunum	
7	Pyloric antrum			

4 Greater curvature, 5 Body, 6 Lesser curvature } of stomach

237 Ileocolic orifice of a dog. The ileum and the ascending colon have been opened to reveal the change in the nature of the mucosal lining.

1	Ileum
2	Caecum
3	Caecal fold
4	Ileocolic orifice and sphincter
5	Accessory ileocaecal fold
6	Caecocolic orifice
7	Ascending colon
8	Lymph follicles

238 Intestinal tract of a cat. The viscera have been removed from the abdomen and arranged to display the ileocolic junction and the simple, uncoiled blind sac of the caecum of a cat.

1 Coils of jejunum
2 Great mesentery
3 Mesenteric lymph nodes
4 Mesenteric arteries and veins
5 Ileum
6 Caecum
7 Ascending colon
8 Transverse colon
9 Descending colon

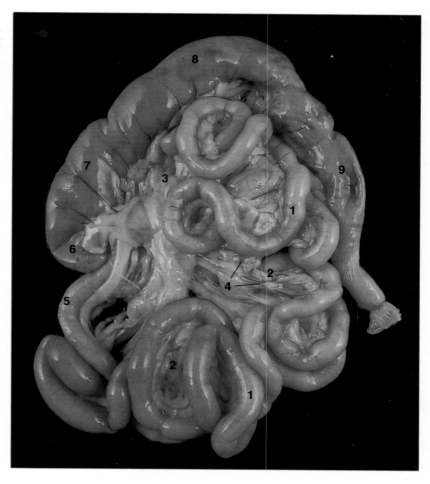

239 Kidney, spleen and liver of a cat.

1 Kidney with capsular veins
2 Renal hilus
3 Parietal surface ⎫
4 Dorsal border ⎬ of spleen
5 Cranial border ⎭
6 Visceral surface ⎫
7 Left lateral lobe ⎪
8 Left medial lobe ⎪
9 Quadrate lobe ⎬ of liver
10 Right medial lobe ⎪
11 Right lateral lobe ⎪
12 Caudate lobe ⎭
13 Caudate process ⎫ of 12
14 Papillary process ⎭
15 Porta
16 Gall bladder
17 Dorsal border of liver

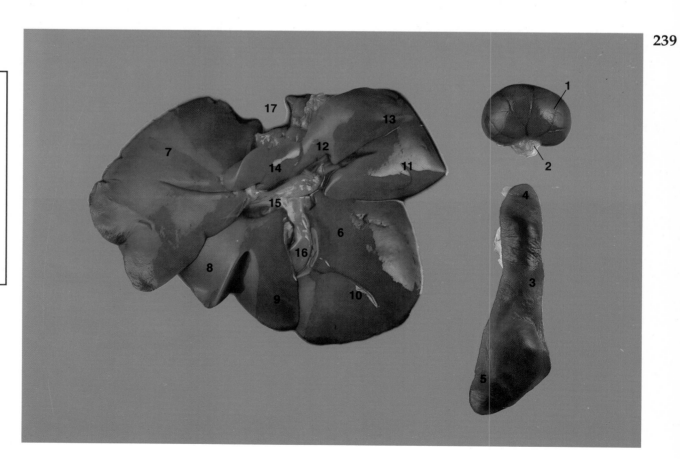

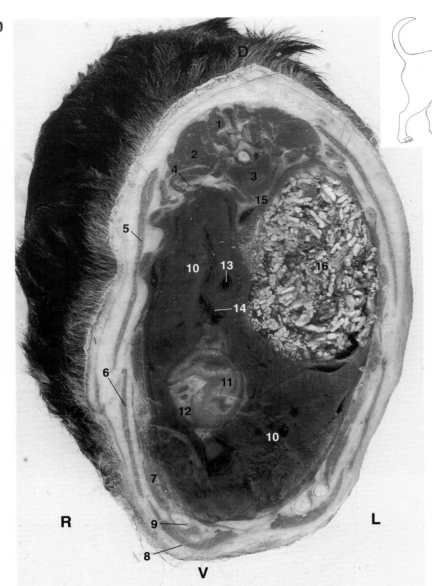

240 Cranial aspect of a transverse section through the abdomen of a dog, at the level of the eleventh thoracic vertebra. Dorsal (D), ventral (V), left (L) and right (R) orientations are indicated.

1	Mm. multifidus thoracis and lumborum
2	Mm. longissimus thoracis and lumborum
3	Eleventh thoracic vertebra
4	Rib
5	M. latissimus dorsi
6	M. obliquus externus abdominis
7	M. intercostalis
8	M. rectus abdominis
9	Costal cartilages
10	Liver
11	Pylorus
12	Pancreas
13	Caudal vena cava
14	Portal vein
15	Aorta
16	Body of stomach (with contents)

241 Cranial face of a transverse section through the abdominal region of a dog, at the level of the first and second lumbar vertebrae. Left (L) and right (R) orientations are indicated.

1	Mm. multifidus thoracis and lumborum	19	Greater omentum
2	Second lumbar vertebra	20	Jejunum
3	First lumbar vertebra	21	Descending duodenum
4	Invertebral disc	22	Pancreas
5	M. psoas major	23	Transverse colon
6	Mm. longissimus thoracis and lumborum	24	Caudate lobe of liver
7	M. latissimus dorsi	25	Right kidney
8	M. iliocostalis	26	Renal hilus
9	Thirteenth (floating) rib	27	Mesenteric lymph nodes
10	M. serratus dorsalis	28	Root of mesentery
11	M. intercostalis	29	Caudal vena cava
12	Twelfth rib and costochondral junction	30	Aorta
13	M. obliquus externus abdominis	31	Cranial mesenteric vein
14	M. obliquus internus abdominis	32	Lumbar lymph nodes
15	M. transversus abdominis	33	Dorsal extremity of spleen
16	M. rectus abdominis	34	Cranial pole of left kidney
17	Eleventh costal cartilage	35	Gastrosplenic ligament
18	Linea alba	36	Splenic vessels
		37	Pancreas
		38	Caudal extremity of spleen
		39	Descending colon

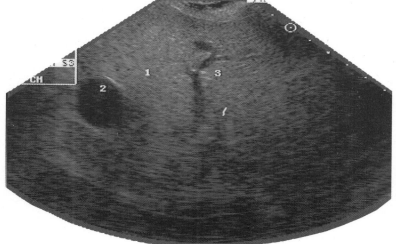

242 Transverse ultrasound scan of the liver of a dog. The gall bladder is seen as a black circular image.

1	Liver
2	Gall bladder
3	Hepatic veins

• Portal veins have walls that give strong echoes, and appear as black structures with bright walls.

243 Longitudinal ultrasound scan of the liver of a dog. The heart can be seen through the diaphragm at depth.

1	Liver
2	Diaphragm
3	Heart
4	Hepatic vein
5	Stomach

244 Lateral radiograph of the abdomen of a dog. A barium enema has been administered to demonstrate the location of the large intestine.

1	First lumbar vertebra
2	Caecum
3	Ascending colon
4	Transverse colon
5	Descending colon
6	Jejunum
7	Rectum
8	Anus
9	Sacrum

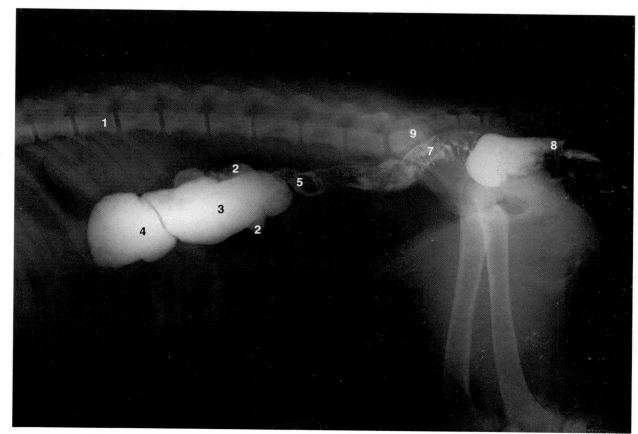

244

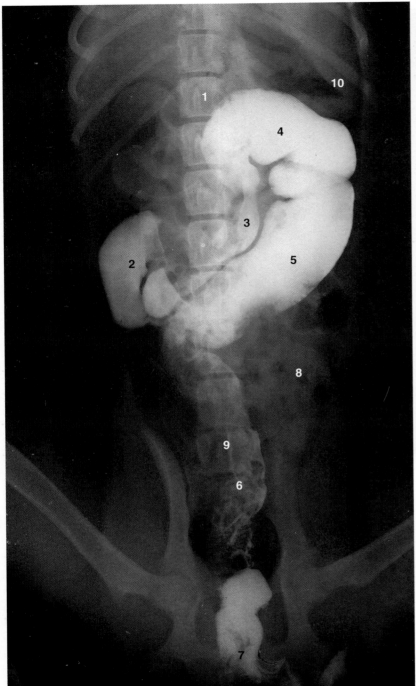

246 Dorsal aspect of the genital tract of a bitch.

1	Ovarian bursa	9	Uterine body
2	Opening of ovarian bursa	10	Uterine artery
3	Suspensory ligament of ovary	11	Urinary bladder
4	Ovarian artery	12	Ureter
5	Mesovarium	13	Vagina
6	Mesometrium	14	Vulva
7	Uterine horn	15	Labia
8	Uterine branch of 4		

245 Ventrodorsal radiograph of the abdomen of a dog. A barium enema has been administered to demonstrate the location of the large intestine.

1	Thirteenth thoracic vertebra	6	Rectum
2	Caecum	7	Anus
3	Ascending colon	8	Jejunum
4	Transverse colon	9	Seventh lumbar vertebra
5	Descending colon	10	Spleen

247 Median section through the caudal abdominal and pelvic cavities of a bitch, showing the left side of the region and the topography of the pelvic contents.

1	Sacrum
2	Seventh lumbar vertebra
3	Descending colon
4	Caudal vena cava
5	Rectum
6	Jejunum
7	Duodenum
8	Uterine horn
9	Uterine body
10	Cervix
11	Urinary bladder
12	Vagina
13	Vestibule
14	Vulva
15	Pubis
16	M. obturatorius internus
17	M. adductor
18	M. rectus abdominis
19	External pudendal artery and vein
20	Superficial inguinal lymph node
21	Inguinal mammary gland
22	Teat
23	Caudal superficial epigastric artery and vein

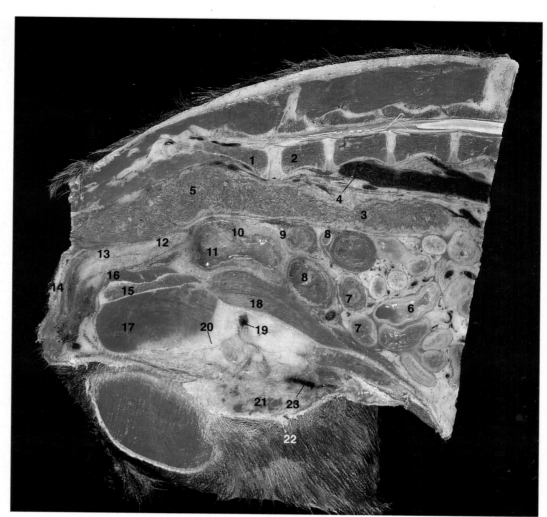

248 Cranial aspect of a transverse section of the trunk of a bitch, at the level of the seventh lumbar vertebra.

1	Wing of ilium
2	Seventh lumbar vertebra
3	M. iliopsoas
4	Internal iliac artery and vein
5	Rectum
6	Uterine body
7	Urinary bladder
8	M. rectus abdominis
9	Mammary gland
10	Femur

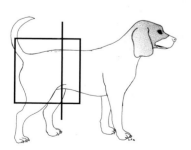

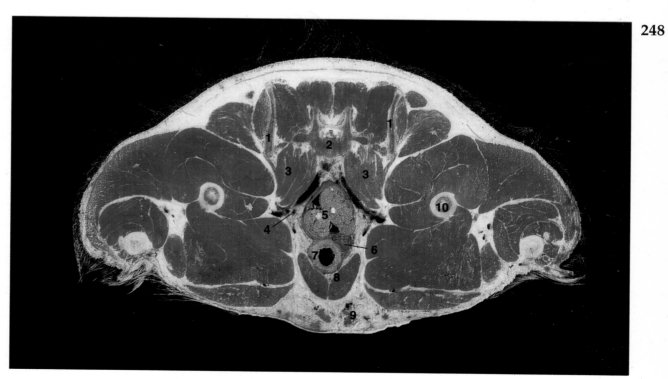

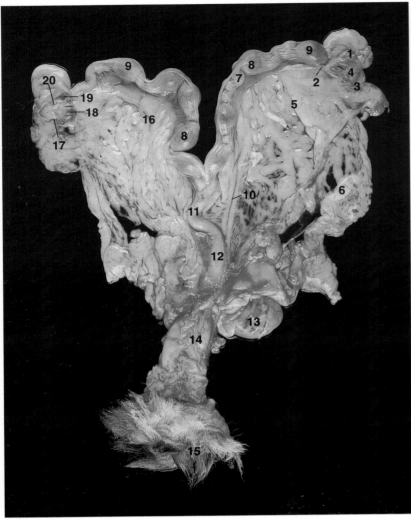

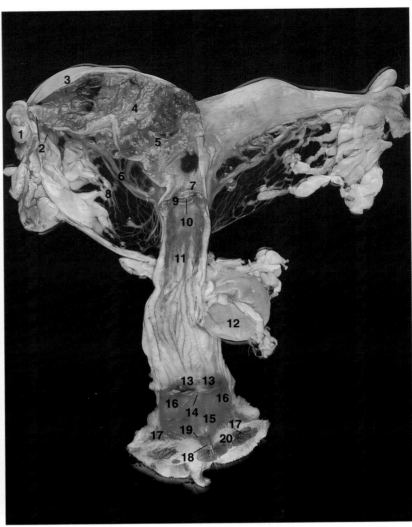

249 Dorsal aspect of the uterus of a pregnant bitch.

1	Suspensory ligament	of ovary	
2	Proper ligament		
3	Mesovarium		
4	Opening of ovarian bursa		
5	Mesometrium (broad ligament)		
6	Round ligament		
7	Uterine horn		
8	Loci of conceptuses		
9	Area of zonary band		
10	Uterine artery and vein		
11	Uterine body		
12	Vagina		
13	Urinary bladder		
14	Vestibule		
15	Vulva		
16	Uterine branch of ovarian artery and vein		
17	Ovarian bursa (opened)		
18	Ovary bearing corpora lutea		
19	Infundibulum		
20	Oviduct		

250 Dorsal aspect of the genital tract of a bitch. The tract, which has been opened dorsally, illustrates an endometrial lining that is typical of a postparturient bitch.

1	Ovary extruded from bursa	10	External uterine orifice
2	Uterine tube	11	Vagina
3	Uterine horn	12	Urinary bladder
4	Endometrium	13	Mucosal folds
5	Area of detached placentation (zonary)	14	External urethral orifice
6	Uterine branch of ovarian artery and vein	15	Vestibule
7	Uterine body	16	Vestibular bulb
8	Mesometrium (broad ligament)	17	M. constrictor vestibuli
9	Cervix	18	Clitoris
		19	Fossa clitoridis
		20	Labia

251 Dorsal aspect of the uterus of a pregnant cat, showing the location of four conceptuses.

1   Ovary with corpora lutea
2   Mesovarium with ovarian artery and vein
3   Gravid left uterine horn
4   Mesometrium
5   Uterine branch of ovarian artery
6   Placental bands seen through myometrium
7   Uterine body
8   Right uterine horn
9   Round ligament
10 Urinary bladder
11 Level of cervix
12 Vagina
13 Vestibule
14 Vulva

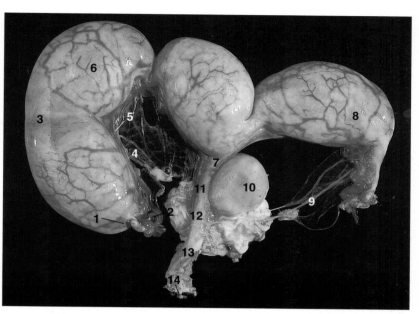

252 Dorsal aspect of the uterus of a pregnant cat. The loculus of the right horn has been opened and the foetus, surrounded by the foetal membranes and zonary placenta, has been displaced. The vulva, vestibule and vagina have been opened dorsally.

1   Zonary placental band surrounding foetus
2   Foetus within foetal membranes
3   Cranium
4   Tail and pelvic limb of foetus
5   Myometrium (stripped of endometrium)
6   Intact loculi
7   Ovary with corpora lutea
8   Vulva
9   Vestibule
10 Fossa clitoridis enclosing clitoris
11 External urethral orifice
12 Vagina
13 Cervix
14 Uterine body

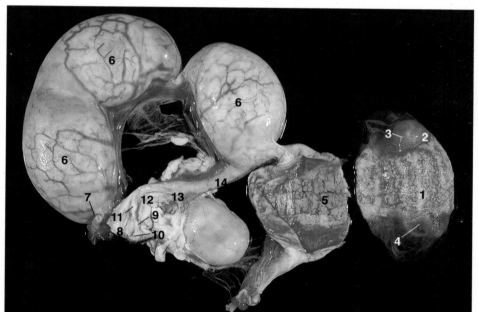

253 Feline foetus with opened foetal membranes and sectioned placental band.

1   Foetus
2   Umbilicus
3   Umbilical vessels
4   Opened foetal membranes
5   Placental band

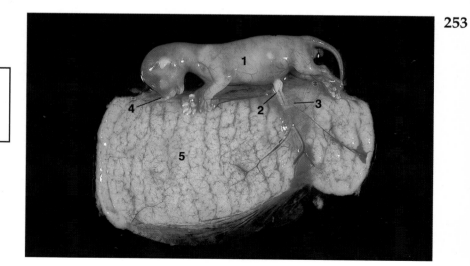

254

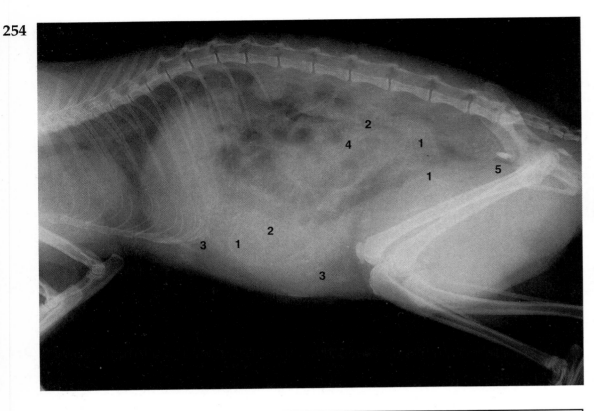

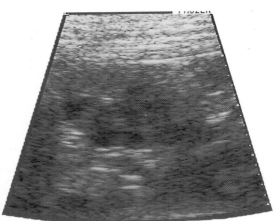

255 Ultrasound scan of the ovary of a bitch, made through the lateral abdominal wall. The muscle layers can be seen at the top of the scan and the ovary occupies the centre of the field. The darkened circular areas on the ovarian surface are follicles.

255

254 Lateral radiograph of the abdomen of a pregnant cat.

1	Foetal skulls	4	Foetal ribs
2	Foetal vertebrae	5	Pelvic inlet
3	Foetal limbs		

256a

256c

256b

256 Ultrasound scans of the uteri of three pregnant bitches, through the ventral abdominal wall.

In **A** (a 28-day pregnancy) the urinary bladder is seen as a circular black area at the top of the scan. The other two circular areas (at 2 o'clock and 10 o'clock) are cross-sectional images of the gravid uterine horns. The conceptuses are seen as grey areas within the horns.

B (a 32-day pregnancy) is a magnified longitudinal scan of a foetus within the uterine horn, with the head to the right. The limb buds are also evident.

C is a scan of the thoracic region of a foetus in late pregnancy. The foetal ribs are evident as strong, white echoes lying in the centre of the field and extending to the left (1). The placentary band can be seen peripheral to this (2).

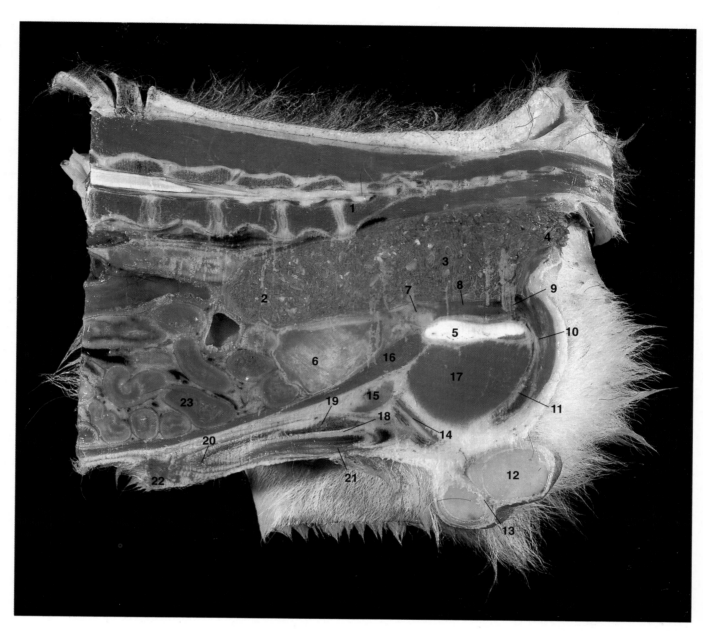

257 Paramedian section of the caudal abdominal and pelvic cavities of a male dog, showing the topography of the pelvic contents and the external genitalia.

1	Sacrum	9	Penile urethra	17	M. adductor
2	Descending colon	10	M. ischiocavernosus	18	Os penis
3	Rectum	11	Corpus cavernosum penis	19	Bulbus glandis
4	Anus	12	Testis	20	Pars longa glandis
5	Pubis	13	Scrotum	21	Penile urethra in ventral groove
6	Urinary bladder	14	Spermatic cord	22	Prepuce
7	Prostate	15	Superficial inguinal lymph node	23	Jejunum
8	Pelvic urethra	16	M. rectus abdominis		

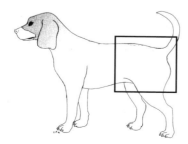

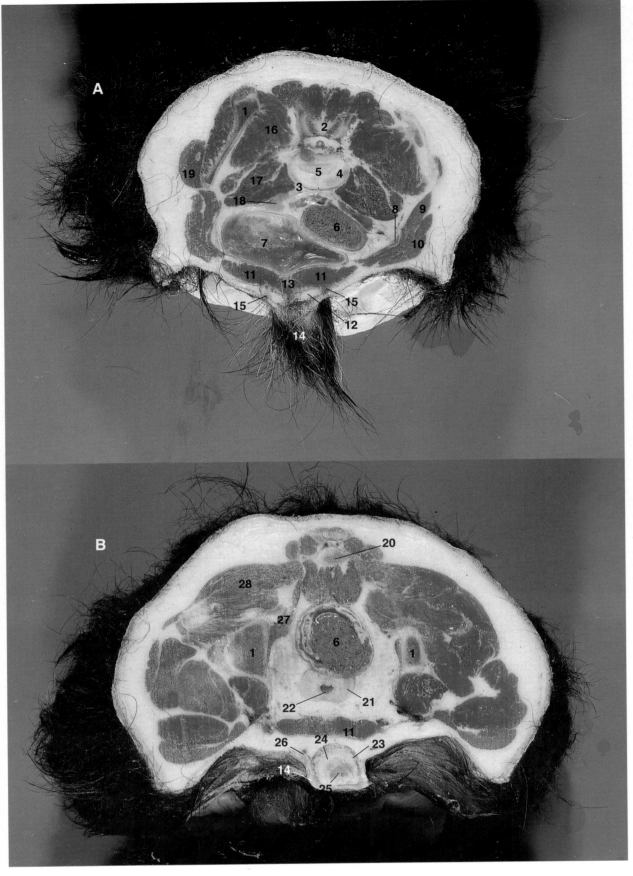

Cranial aspect of transverse sections through the seventh lumbar (A) and first caudal (B) vertebrae of a male dog, showing the topography of the pelvic contents.

1	Ilium
2	Seventh lumbar vertebra
3	Intervertebral disc
4	Annulus fibrosus
5	Nucleus pulposus
6	Rectum
7	Urinary bladder
8	M. transversus abdominis
9	M. obliquus internus abdominis
10	M. obliquus externus abdominis
11	M. rectus abdominis
12	M. protractor preputii
13	Linea alba
14	Prepuce
15	Preputial branches of external pudendal artery
16	Mm. iliocostalis and longissimus lumborum
17	Mm. iliacus and psoas major
18	Hypogastric lymph node
19	M. tensor fasciae latae
20	First caudal vertebra
21	Prostate gland
22	Pelvic urethra
23	Bulbus glandis of penis
24	Os penis
25	Penile urethra
26	Superficial branch of dorsal artery of penis
27	M. coccygeus
28	Gluteal muscle mass

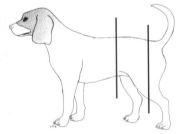

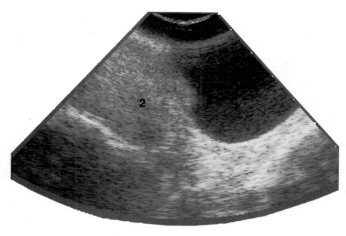

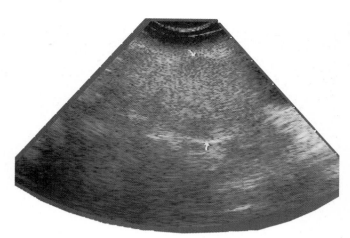

259 Ultrasound scan through the ventral abdominal wall of a male dog, made in the prepubic location. The urinary bladder can be seen with the prostate immediately adjacent to it.

260 Caudal ultrasound scan through the ventral abdominal wall of a male dog, made in the prepubic location. The bilobed nature of the prostate, which is in cross section, can be seen. Arrows indicate the outline of one lobe.

1	Urinary bladder	2	Prostate gland

261 Caudal aspect of the perineum of a bitch.

1	M. sacrocaudalis ventralis lateralis
2	M. rectococcygeus
3	M. sphincter ani externus
4	M. coccygeus
5	M. levator ani
6	Anus
7	Ischiatic tuberosity
8	M. obturatorius internus
9	M. ischiourethralis
10	M. constrictor vestibuli
11	M. constrictor vulvae
12	Labia
13	Vulva
14	M. biceps femoris
15	M. semitendinosus
16	M. semimembranosus
17	M. gracilis
18	Internal pudendal artery and vein, and pudendal nerve
19	Caudal rectal artery and vein
20	Perineal artery and vein
21	Artery and vein of vestibular bulb

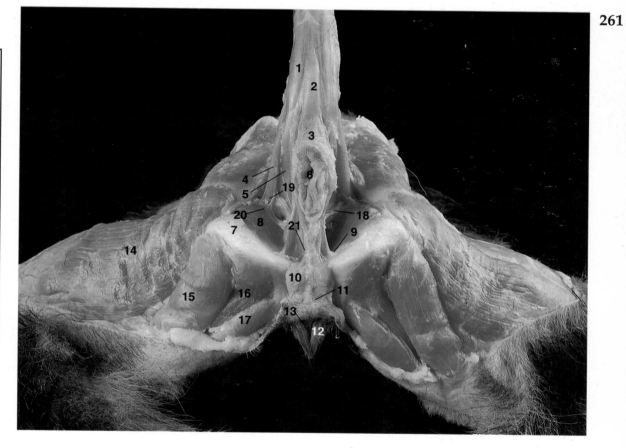

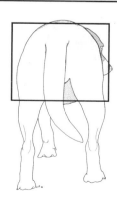

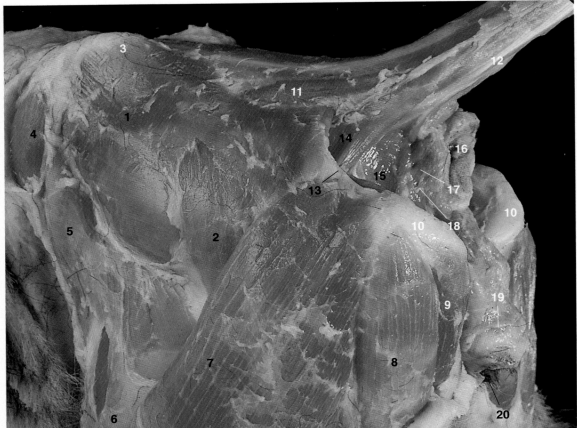

262 Caudolateral aspect of the perineum and external genitalia of a bitch.

1	M. gluteus medius
2	M. gluteus superficialis
3	Cranial dorsal iliac spine
4	M. sartorius
5	M. tensor fascia latae
6	Fascia lata
7	M. biceps femoris
8	M. semitendinosus
9	M. semimembranosus
10	Ischiatic tuberosity
11	Mm. intertransversarii dorsales caudales
12	Mm. intertransversarii ventrales caudales
13	Sacrotuberous ligament
14	M. coccygeus
15	M. levator ani
16	Anus
17	M. sphincter ani externus
18	Fibres from first and second caudal spinal nerves
19	M. constrictor vulvae
20	Vulva

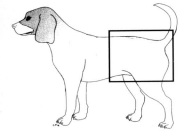

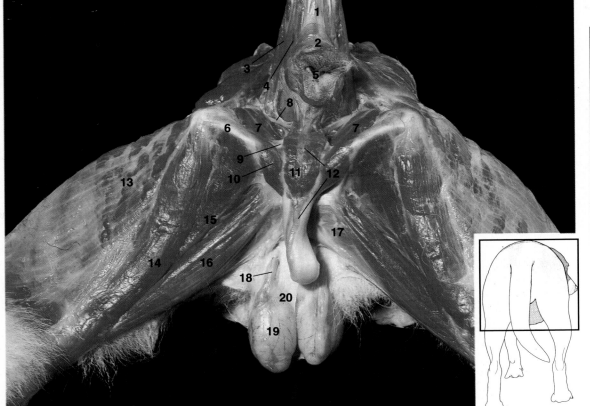

263 Caudal aspect of the perineum and external genitalia of a male dog.

1	M. rectococcygeus
2	M. sphincter ani externus
3	M. coccygeus
4	M. levator ani
5	Anus
6	Ischiatic tuberosity
7	M. obturatorius internus
8	Internal pudendal artery and vein, and pudendal nerve
9	M. ischiourethralis
10	M. ischiocavernosus
11	M. bulbospongiosus
12	M. retractor penis
13	M. biceps femoris
14	M. semitendinosus
15	M. semimembranosus
16	M. gracilis
17	M. adductor
18	Spermatic cord
19	Testis within parietal vaginal tunic
20	External spermatic fascia

264 Caudolateral aspect of the perineum of a male dog.

1 Cranial dorsal iliac spine
2 M. gluteus medius
3 M. gluteus superficialis
4 M. sartorius
5 M. tensor fasciae latae
6 Greater trochanter
7 M. biceps femoris
8 M. semitendinosus
9 M. semimembranosus
10 M. gracilis
11 Ischiatic tuberosity
12 Sacrotuberous ligament
13 Mm. intertransversarii dorsales caudales
14 Mm. intertransversarii ventrales caudales
15 M. coccygeus
16 M. levator ani
17 Anus
18 M. sphincter ani externus
19 Position of anal sac (deep to 18)
20 M. rectococcygeus
21 Fibres from first and second caudal spinal nerves
22 M. retractor penis
23 M. bulbospongiosus
24 M. ischiocavernosus
25 M. ischiourethralis
26 Body of penis
27 Corpus spongiosum penis
28 M. obturatorius internus
29 Internal pudendal artery giving origin to dorsal artery of penis and ventral perineal artery
30 Caudal rectal artery
31 Pudendal nerve

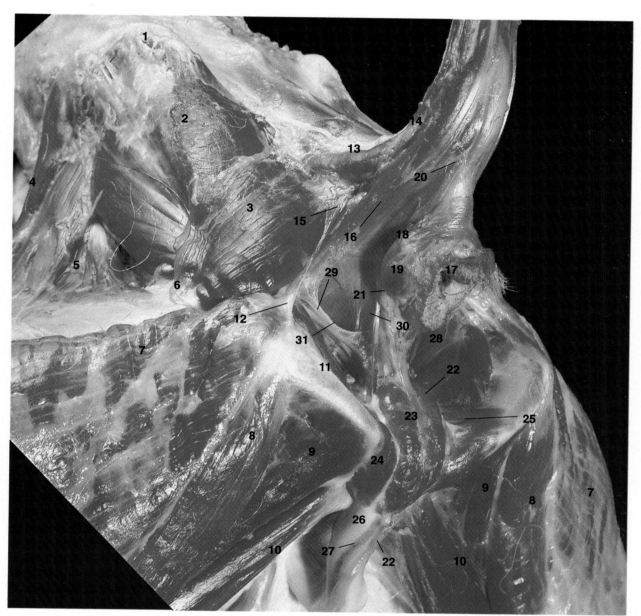

265 Dorsal (A) and ventral (B) aspect of the os penis of a dog.

1 Cranial extremity
2 Caudal extremity (proximal)
3 Ventral groove

- Note the ventral groove which encloses the urethra in life. Urethral obstruction commonly occurs at the proximal end of this groove.

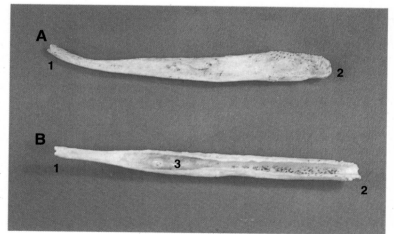

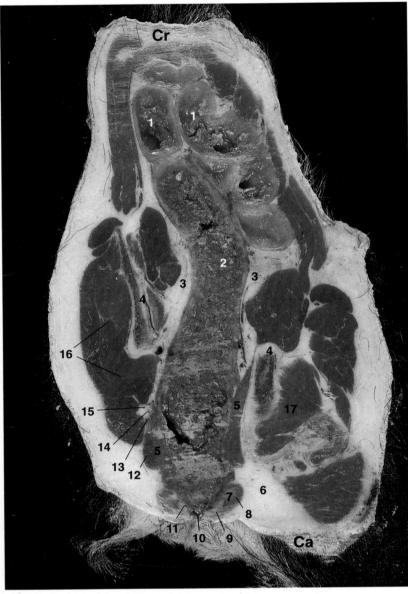

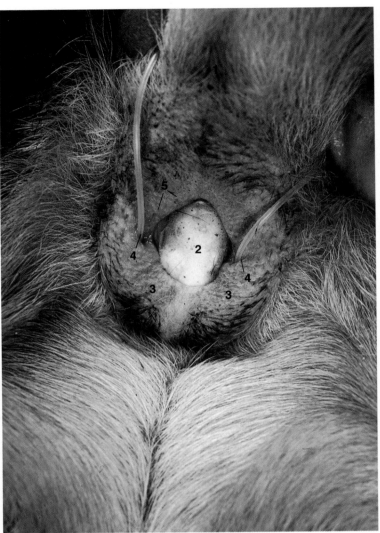

267 Caudal aspect of the anal region of a dog. The ducts of the anal sacs have been cannulated.

1	Tail		(cannulated)
2	Anus (with cotton plug)	5	Elevations for openings of
3	Cutaneous zone		circumanal glands
4	Opening of anal sac		

266 Dorsal aspect of a section made in the dorsal plane through the anus and pelvic cavity of a dog, showing the topography of the rectum and the muscles of the pelvic diaphragm. Orientation cranially (Cr) and caudally (Ca) is indicated.

1	Descending colon	10	Anal opening
2	Rectum	11	M. sphincter ani internus
3	Pelvic inlet	12	M. coccygeus
4	Ilium	13	Sacrotuberous ligament
5	M. levator ani	14	Ischiatic nerve
6	Fat (in ischiorectal fossa)	15	Caudal gluteal artery and vein
7	Anal sac	16	Gluteal muscle
8	M. sphincter ani externus	17	Mm. gemelli
9	Circumanal glands		

- Observe the relative proximity of the ischiatic nerve and the sacrotuberous ligament: in the repair of a perineal hernia, the ligament is used as an anchor point for suturing the muscles of the pelvic diaphragm (M. coccygeus and M. levator ani) and entrapment of the ischiatic nerve in the suture is a potential hazard.

268 Radiograph of the lateral aspect of the thorax and abdomen of a dog. Barium has been administered by mouth, and is seen in the upper digestive tract.

1	Oesophagus
2	Heart
3	Diaphragm
4	Thirteenth (floating) rib
5	Thirteenth vertebra
6	Fundus ⎫
7	Body ⎬ of stomach
8	Pyloric antrum ⎭
9	Liver
10	Spleen
11	Duodenum
12	Jejunum
13	Caecum
14	Abdominal wall

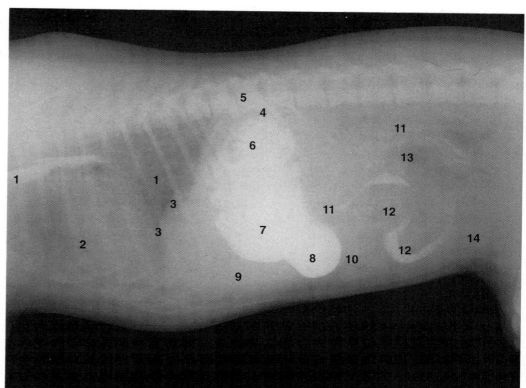

269 Ventrodorsal radiograph of the abdominal region of a dog in dorsal recumbency. Barium is lying intermingled with air in the stomach. The duodenum is outlined by barium filling, demonstrating the typical villous lining.

1	Diaphragm
2	Liver
3	Thirteenth (floating) rib
4	Cardia
5	Fundus (with barium) ⎫
6	Body (with air and barium) ⎬ of stomach
7	Pyloric antrum ⎭
8	Pylorus
9	Descending duodenum
10	Ascending duodenum
11	Jejunum
12	Ileum

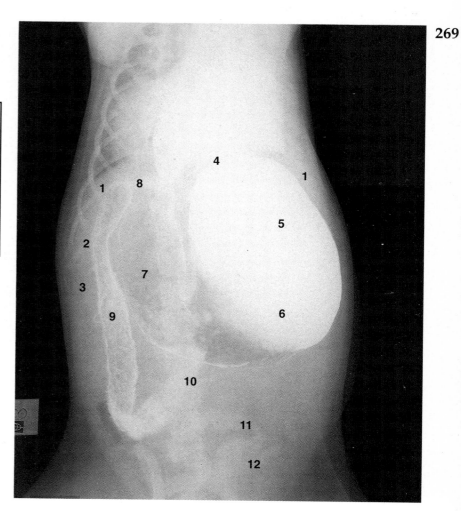

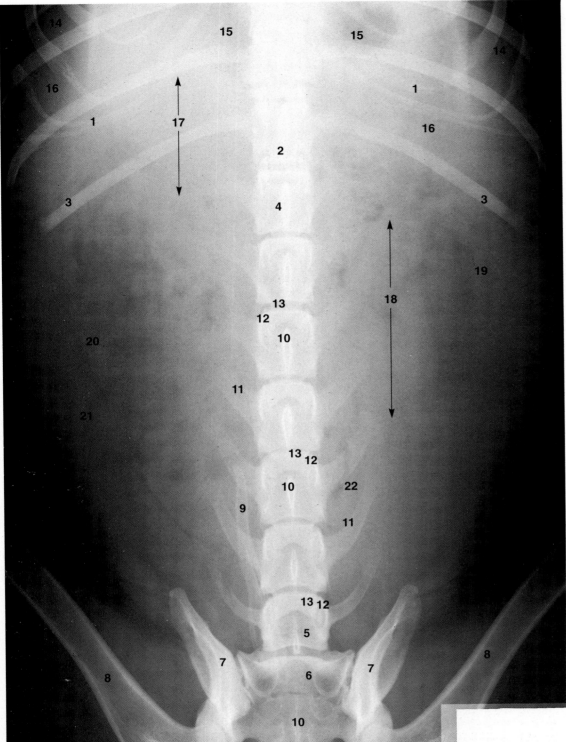

270 Radiograph of the abdominal
region of a male dog in
ventrodorsal positioning.

1	Costal arch
2	Thirteenth thoracic vertebra
3	Thirteenth (oating) rib
4	First lumbar vertebra
5	Seventh lumbar vertebra
6	Sacrum
7	Ilium
8	Femur
9	Os penis
10	Spinous process
11	Transverse process
12	Cranial articular process and mamillary process
13	Caudal articular process
14	Diaphragm
15	Stomach
16	Liver
17	Right kidney
18	Left kidney
19	Spleen
20	Jejunum
21	Caecum
22	Descending colon

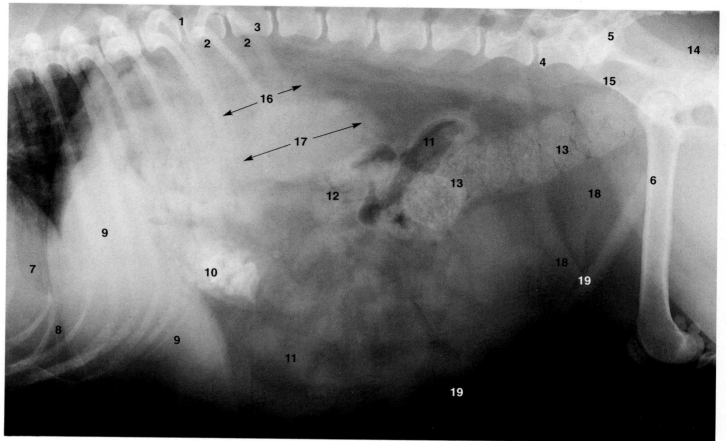

271 Radiograph of the abdominal region of a male dog in lateral recumbency.

1	Thirteenth thoracic vertebra	12	Region of ileocolic and caecolic junction
2	Thirteenth (floating) rib	13	Descending colon
3	First lumbar vertebra	14	Rectum
4	Seventh lumbar vertebra	15	Wing of ilium
5	Sacrum	16	Right kidney (arrows)
6	Femur	17	Left kidney (arrows)
7	Heart	18	Urinary bladder (distended, intra-abdominal)
8	Diaphragm	19	Ventral abdominal wall
9	Liver		
10	Stomach		
11	Jejunum		

7 Pelvic Limb

Working from the proximal pelvic region distally to the pes, the osteological details of each area of the pelvic limb are illustrated using bones, displayed both singly and in an articulated form, and radiographs. The relevant musculature is then exhibited. Contrast arteriograms and venograms are used to give an overview of the vascular supply, while nerve trunks are named where they appear in the dissected specimens.

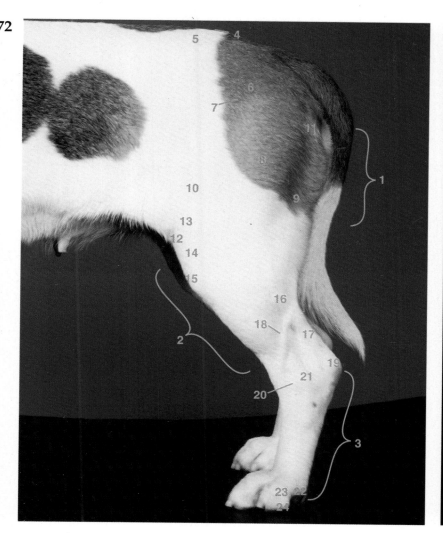

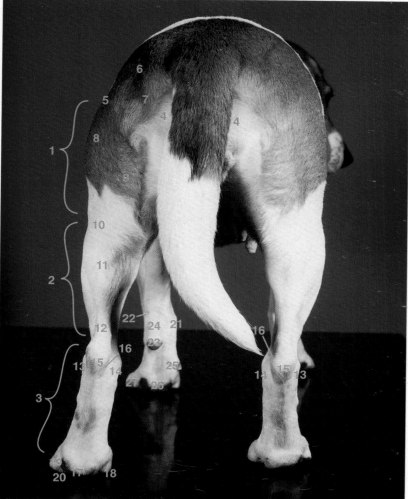

272 Lateral aspect of the left pelvic limb of a standing live dog, demonstrating palpable landmarks.

1	Femoral region (thigh)	14	Stifle joint
2	Crus	15	Tibial tuberosity
3	Pes	16	M. gastrocnemius
4	Median crest of sacrum	17	Tendo calcaneus communis (Achilles)
5	Cranial dorsal iliac spine	18	Lateral saphenous vein (site of intravenous injection)
6	Greater trochanter		
7	Level of hip joint	19	Calcaneal tuberosity
8	M. biceps femoris	20	Tarsal joint (hock)
9	M. semitendinosus	21	Lateral malleolus of fibula
10	M. quadriceps femoris	22	Metatarsal pad
11	Ischiatic tuberosity	23	Fifth digit
12	Patella	24	Digital pad
13	Lateral epicondyle of femur		

273 Caudal aspect of a standing live dog, demonstrating palpable landmarks. The palmar aspect of the manus of the thoracic limb is also shown.

1	Femoral region (thigh)	14	Medial malleolus of tibia
2	Crus	15	Calcaneal tuberosity
3	Pes	16	Tarsal joint (hock)
4	Perineum	17	Metatarsal pad
5	Greater trochanter	18	Second digit
6	Gluteal muscle mass	19	Fifth digit
7	Ischiatic tuberosity	20	Digital pad
8	M. biceps femoris	21	Medial styloid process of radius
9	M. semitendinosus	22	Carpal joint
10	Stifle joint	23	Carpal pad
11	M. gastrocnemius and M. flexor digitorum superficialis	24	Accessory carpal bone
		25	First digit (dew claw)
12	Tendo calcaneus communis (Achilles)	26	Metacarpal pad
		27	Fifth digit
13	Lateral malleolus of fibula		

(21–27 labelled as "thoracic limb")

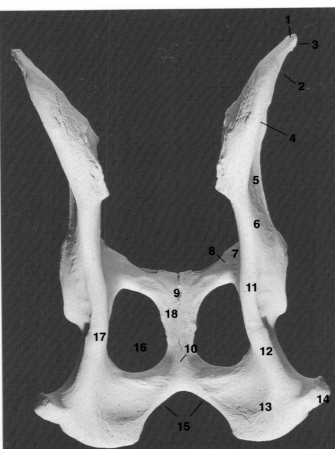

274 Dorsal aspect of the fused ossa coxae of a dog.

1	Iliac crest
2	Wing of ilium
3	Cranial dorsal iliac spine
4	Caudal dorsal iliac spine
5	Body of ilium
6	Greater ischiatic notch
7	Iliopubic eminence
8	Pecten of pubic bone
9	Symphysis pubis
10	Symphysis ischii
11	Ischiatic spine
12	Lesser ischiatic notch
13	Ischiatic table
14	Ischiatic tuberosity
15	Ischiatic arch
16	Obturator foramen
17	Grooves for M. obturatorius internus
18	Pubis

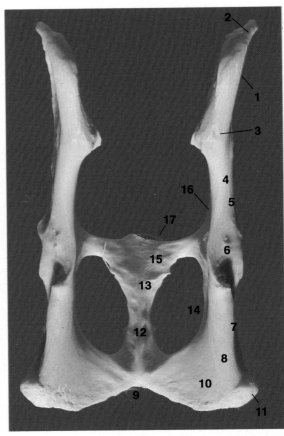

275 Dorsal aspect of the fused ossa coxae of a cat.

1	Wing of ilium
2	Cranial dorsal iliac spine
3	Caudal dorsal iliac spine
4	Body of ilium
5	Greater ischiatic notch
6	Ischiatic spine
7	Lesser ischiatic notch
8	Ischium
9	Ischiatic arch
10	Ischiatic table
11	Ischiatic tuberosity
12	Symphysis ischii } symphysis pelvis
13	Symphysis pubis
14	Obturator foramen
15	Pubis
16	Arcuate line
17	Pecten of pubic bone

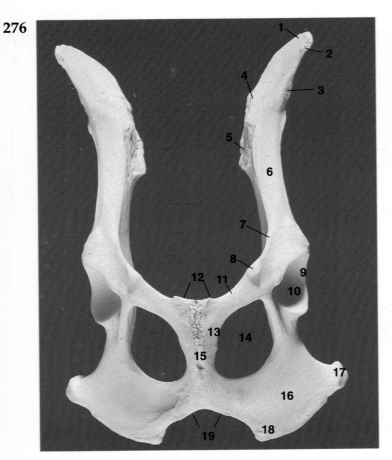

276 Ventral aspect of the fused ossa coxae of a dog.

1	Iliac crest	11	Pecten of pubic bone
2	Cranial ventral iliac spine	12	Pubic tubercle
3	Caudal ventral iliac spine	13	Pubis
4	Iliac tuberosity	14	Obturator foramen
5	Auricular surface	15	Symphysis pelvis
6	Body of ilium	16	Ischium
7	Arcuate line	17	Ischiatic tuberosity
8	Iliopubic eminence	18	Medial angle of 17
9	Lunate surface of acetabulum	19	Ischiatic arch
10	Acetabular fossa		

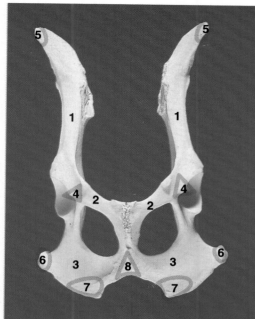

277 Ventral aspect of the fused ossa coxae of a dog, showing the centres of ossification.

1	Body of ilium
2	Body of pubis
3	Body of ischium
4	Acetabular bone
5	Iliac crest
6	Ischiatic tuberosity
7	Ischiatic arch
8	Symphysis

278 Ventral aspect of the fused ossa coxae of a cat.

1	Iliac crest
2	Cranial ventral iliac spine
3	Caudal ventral iliac spine
4	Auricular surface
5	Body of ilium
6	Arcuate line
7	Acetabular fossa
8	Lunate surface of acetabulum
9	Body of ischium
10	Ischiatic tuberosity
11	Obturator foramen
12	Ischiatic arch
13	Symphysis pelvis
14	Pubis
15	Pubic tubercle
16	Pecten of pubic bone
17	Iliopubic eminence

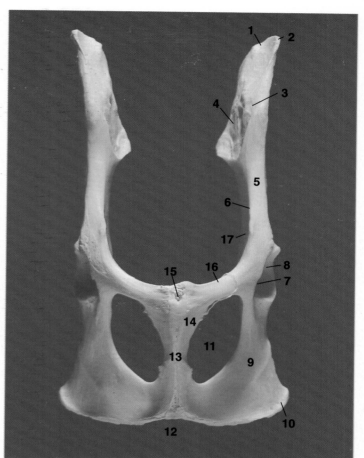

279 Lateral aspect of the left os coxae of a cat.

1	Cranial dorsal iliac spine
2	Caudal dorsal iliac spine
3	Body of ilium
4	Greater ischiatic notch
5	Ischiatic spine
6	Acetabular fossa
7	Lunate surface of acetabulum
8	Acetabular incisura
9	Lesser ischiatic notch
10	Body of ischium
11	Ischiatic tuberosity
12	Obturator foramen
13	Pubis
14	Pubic tubercle
15	Pecten of pubic bone
16	Iliopubic eminence
17	Cranial ventral iliac spine
18	Caudal ventral iliac spine

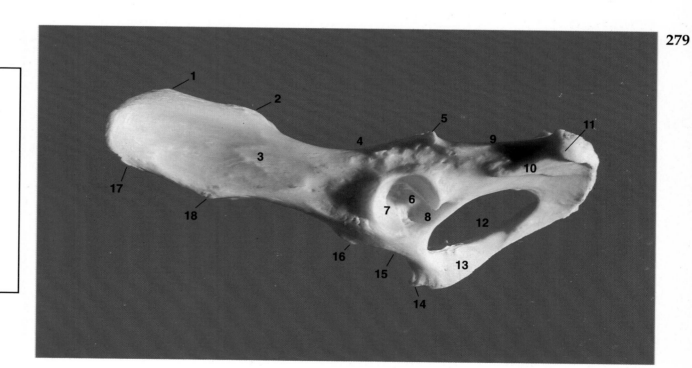

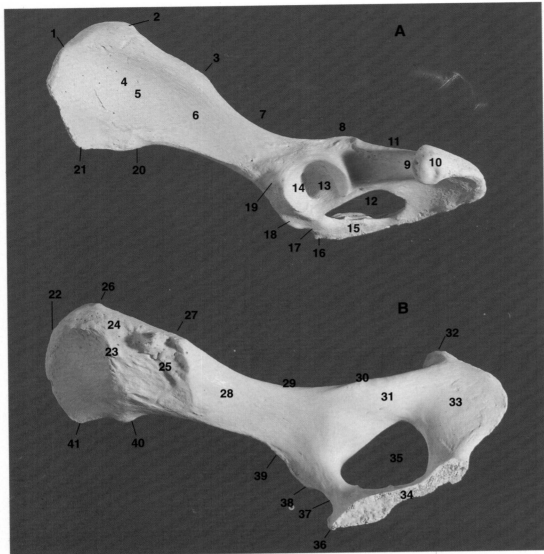

280 Lateral aspect of the left os coxae (A) and medial aspect of the right os coxae (B) of a dog.

1	Iliac crest
2	Cranial dorsal iliac spine
3	Caudal dorsal iliac spine
4	Wing
5	Gluteal surface } of ilium
6	Body
7	Greater ischiatic notch
8	Ischiatic spine
9	Ischium
10	Ischiatic tuberosity
11	Lesser ischiatic notch
12	Obturator foramen
13	Acetabular fossa
14	Lunate surface of acetabulum
15	Pubis
16	Pubic tubercle
17	Pecten of pubic bone
18	Iliopubic eminence
19	Tuberosity for M. rectus femoris
20	Caudal ventral iliac spine
21	Cranial ventral iliac spine
22	Iliac tuberosity
23	Sacroiliac joint
24	Iliac tuberosity
25	Auricular surface
26	Cranial dorsal iliac spine
27	Caudal dorsal iliac spine
28	Body of ilium
29	Greater ischiatic notch
30	Ischiatic spine
31	Grooves for M. obturatorius internus
32	Ischiatic tuberosity
33	Ischiatic table
34	Symphysis pelvis
35	Obturator foramen
36	Pubic tubercle
37	Pectin of pubic bone
38	Iliopubic eminence
39	Arcuate line
40	Caudal ventral iliac spine
41	Cranial ventral iliac spine

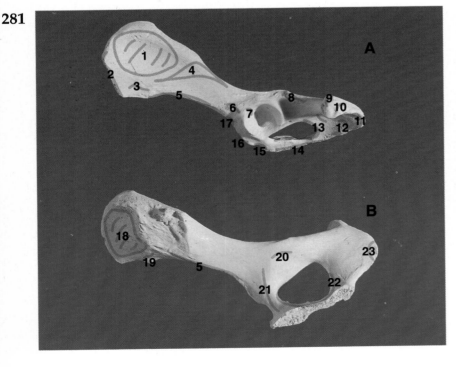

281 Lateral aspect of the left os coxae (A) and medial aspect of the right os coxae (B) of a dog, showing areas of muscle attachment.

1	Middle gluteal	13	Obturatorius externus
2	Sartorius	14	Adductor and gracilis
3	Tensor fasciae latae	15	Rectus abdominis
4	Deep gluteal	16	Pectineus
5	Iliacus	17	Psoas minor
6	Rectus femoris	18	Iliocostalis and longissimus lumborum
7	Articularis coxae	19	Quadratus lumborum
8	Gemelli	20	Coccygeus
9	Biceps femoris	21	Levator ani
10	Semitendinosus	22	Obturatorius internus
11	Semimembranosus	23	Ischiocavernosus
12	Quadratus femoris		

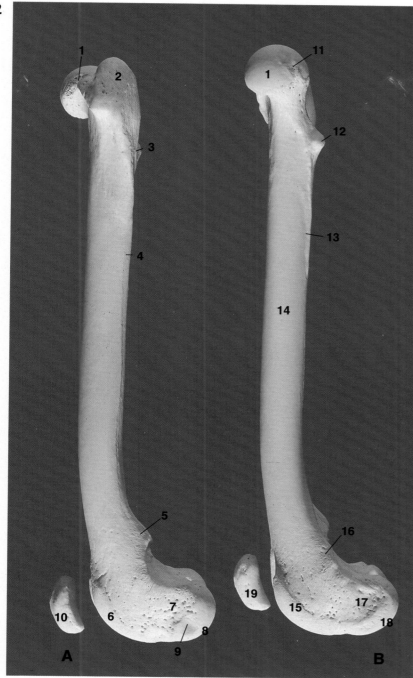

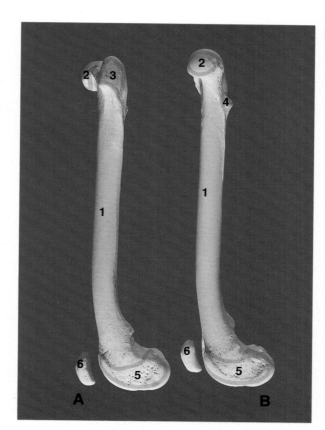

283 Lateral aspect of the left femur (A) and medial aspect of the right femur (B) of a dog, showing the centres of ossification.

1	Body of femur
2	Proximal
3	Greater trochanter
4	Lesser trochanter
5	Distal
6	Patella

282 Lateral aspect of the left femur (A) and medial aspect of the right femur (B) of a dog.

1	Head	11	Fovea
2	Greater trochanter	12	Lesser trochanter
3	Third trochanter (rudimentary)	13	Medial lip
4	Lateral lip	14	Body
5	Lateral supracondylar tuberosity	15	Medial trochlear ridge
6	Lateral trochlear ridge	16	Medial supracondylar tuberosity
7	Lateral epicondyle	17	Medial epicondyle
8	Lateral condyle	18	Medial condyle
9	Extensor fossa	19	Patella
10	Patella		

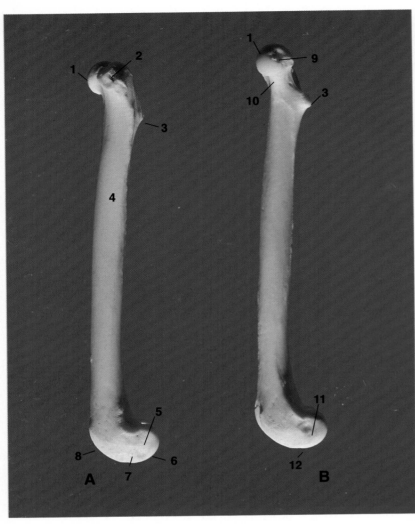

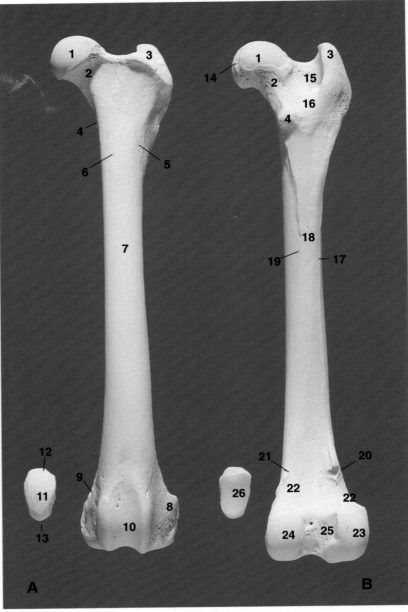

284 Lateral aspect of the left femur (A) and medial aspect of the right femur (B) of a cat.

1	Head	7	Extensor fossa
2	Greater trochanter	8	Trochlea
3	Lesser trochanter	9	Fovea
4	Body	10	Neck
5	Lateral epicondyle	11	Medial epicondyle
6	Lateral condyle	12	Medial condyle

285 Cranial aspect of the left femur (A) and caudal aspect of the right femur (B) of a dog. The cranial and caudal aspects of the patella are also displayed.

1	Head	15	Trochanteric fossa
2	Neck	16	Intertrochanteric crest
3	Greater trochanter	17	Lateral lip
4	Lesser trochanter	18	Roughened face (facies aspera)
5	Line of M. vastus lateralis	19	Medial lip
6	Line of M. vastus medialis	20	Lateral supracondylar tuberosity
7	Body	21	Medial supracondylar tuberosity
8	Lateral epicondyle	22	Area of articulation of sesamoids
9	Medial epicondyle		(fabellae)
10	Trochlea	23	Lateral condyle
11	Patella	24	Medial condyle
12	Base	25	Intercondylar fossa
13	Apex	26	Articular surface of patella
14	Fovea		

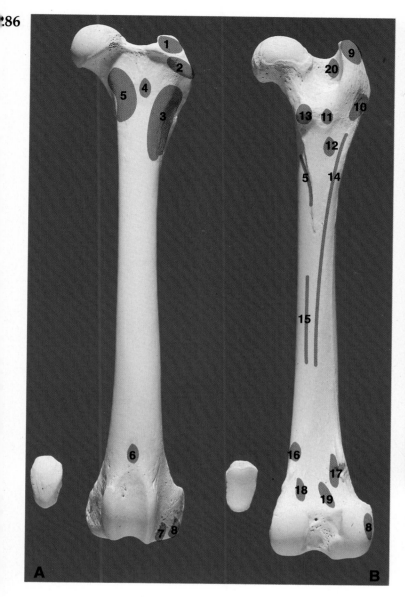

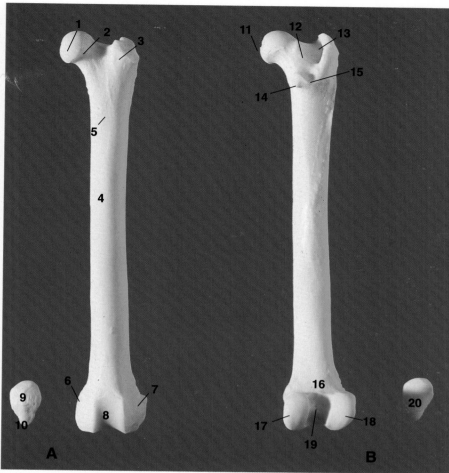

286 Cranial aspect of the left femur (A) and caudal aspect of the right femur (B) of a dog, showing areas of muscle attachment.

287 Cranial aspect (A) of the left femur and caudal aspect (B) of the right femur of a cat.

1	Gluteus medius
2	Gluteus profundus
3	Vastus lateralis and intermedius
4	Articularis coxae
5	Vastus medialis
6	Articularis genus
7	Flexor digitorum longus
8	Popliteus
9	Piriformis and gluteus medius
10	Gluteus superficialias
11	Quadratus femoris
12	Adductor longus
13	Iliopsoas
14	Adductor magnus and brevis
15	Pectineus
16	Semimembranosus
17	Lateral head } of
18	Medial head } Gastrocnemius
19	Flexor digitorum superficialis
20	Gemelli and obturatorius internus and externus

1	Head
2	Neck
3	Greater trochanter
4	Body
5	Line of M. vastus lateralis
6	Medial epicondyle
7	Lateral epicondyle
8	Trochlea
9	Base } of patella
10	Apex } of patella
11	Fovea
12	Trochanteric fossa
13	Greater trochanter
14	Lesser trochanter
15	Intertrochanteric crest
16	Popliteal surface
17	Medial condyle
18	Lateral condyle
19	Intercondylar fossa
20	Articular surface of patella

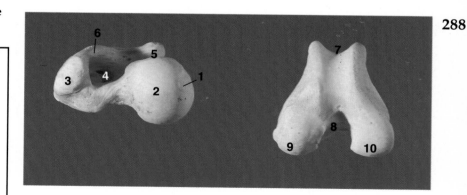

288 Proximal and distal extremities of the femur of a dog.

1	Fovea	6	Intertrochanteric crest
2	Head	7	Trochlea
3	Greater trochanter	8	Intercondylar fossa
4	Trochanteric fossa	9	Lateral condyle
5	Lesser trochanter	10	Medial condyle

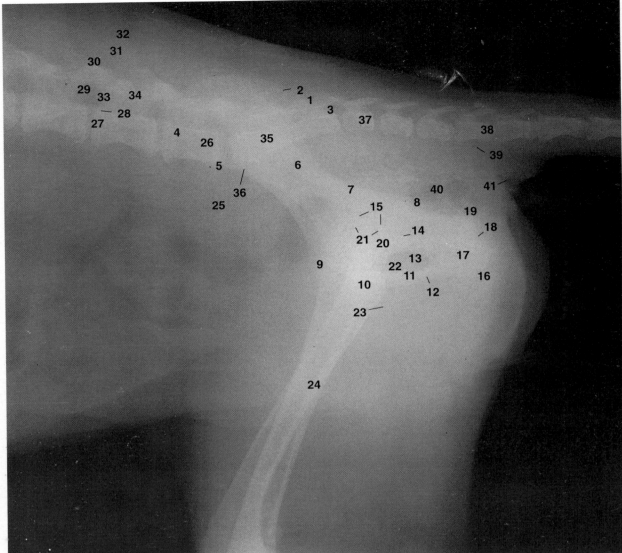

289 Lateral radiograph of the pelvic region of a bitch.

1	Wing of ilium
2	Cranial dorsal iliac spine
3	Caudal dorsal iliac spine
4	Cranial ventral iliac spine
5	Caudal ventral iliac spine
6	Body of ilium
7	Greater ischiatic notch
8	Ischiatic spine
9	Iliopectineal eminence
10	Pecten of pubis
11	Pubis
12	Symphysis pelvis
13	Obturator foramen
14	Acetabular notch
15	Acetabulum
16	Ischiatic arch
17	Ischiatic body
18	Ischiatic tuberosity
19	Lesser ischiatic notch
20	Head of femur
21	Hip joint
22	Greater trochanter
23	Lesser trochanter
24	Body of femur
25	Descending colon
26	Seventh lumbar vertebra
27	Body of sixth lumbar vertebra
28	Transverse process
29	Accessory process
30	Caudal articular process
31	Cranial articular process
32	Spinous process
33	Intervertebral foramen
34	Vertebral canal
35	Wing of sacrum
36	Promontory
37	First caudal vertebra
38	Fifth caudal vertebra
39	Haemal arch
40	Rectum
41	Anus

290 Ventrodorsal radiograph of the pelvis of a male dog.

1 Wing } of ilium
2 Body }
3 Dorsal border
4 Ventral border
5 Caudal ventral iliac spine
6 Cranial ventral iliac spine
7 Iliac crest
8 Acetabular branch of pubis
9 Pecten of pubis
10 Iliopectineal eminence
11 Symphyseal branch of pubis
12 Symphyseal branch of ischium
13 Ischiatic table
14 Ischiatic tuberosity
15 Body of ischium
16 Lesser ischiatic notch
17 Ischiatic arch
18 Obturator foramen
19 Ischiatic spine
20 Dorsal acetabular border
21 Ventral acetabular border
22 Acetabular fossa and incisura
23 Cranial edge } of acetabular
24 Caudal edge } image
25 Head } of femur
26 Neck }
27 Greater trochanter
28 Trochanteric fossa
29 Lesser trochanter
30 Body of femur
31 Descending colon
32 Body of seventh lumbar
   vertebra
33 Spinous process
34 Transverse process
35 Wing of sacrum
36 Rectum
37 Body } of fifth caudal
38 Transverse } vertebra
   process
39 Outline of scrotum
40 Outline of penis
41 Os penis overlying caudal
   vertebrae and sacrum

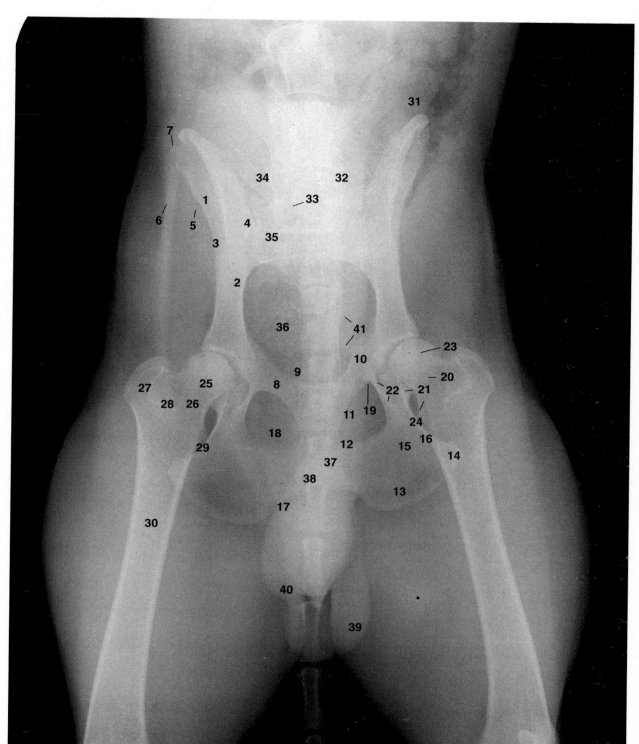

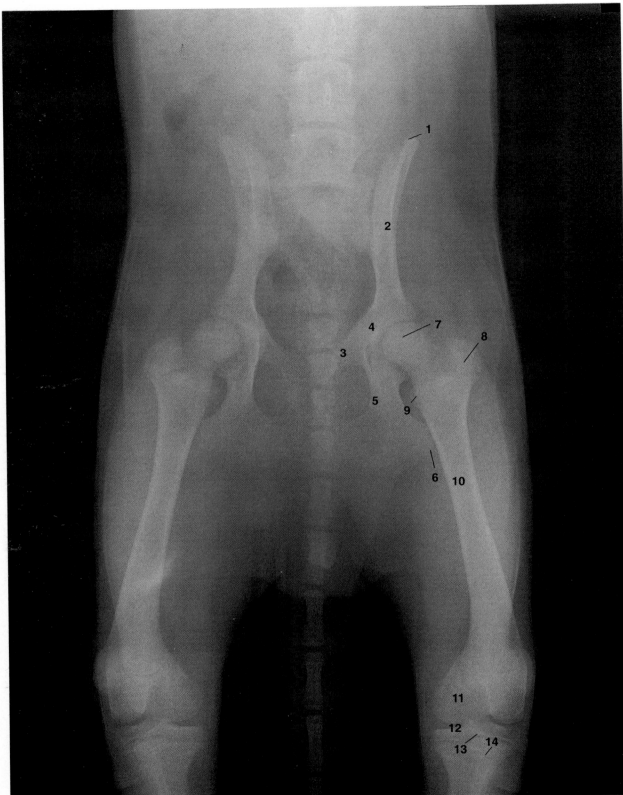

1	Iliac crest
2	Body of ilium
3	Pubis
4	Acetabular bone
5	Body of ischium
6	Ischiatic tuberosity
7	Head of femur
8	Greater trochanter
9	Lesser trochanter
10	Body of femur
11	Distal femoral epiphysis
12	Proximal tibial epiphysis
13	Proximal fibular epiphysis
14	Tibial tuberosity

292 Lateral aspect of the pelvic and thigh regions of the left pelvic limb of a dog. The skin has been removed to reveal the superficial muscles.

1 Dorsal iliac spine
2 Sacrum
3 Caudal vertebrae
4 Mm. intertransversarii dorsales caudalis
5 Mm. intertransversarii ventrales caudalis
6 Sacrotuberous ligament
7 Ischiatic tuberosity
8 Greater trochanter
9 M. gluteus medius
10 M. gluteus superficialis
11 M. sartorius
12 M. tensor fasciae latae
13 M. biceps femoris
14 M. semitendinosus
15 M. semimembranosus
16 Fascia lata extending to stifle
17 Continuation of M. biceps femoris
18 Patella in trochlear groove
19 Lateral epicondyle of femur
20 Tibial tuberosity
21 Patellar ligament
22 M. tibialis cranialis
23 Lateral saphenous vein
24 Medial saphenous vein

• This is the approach for exposing the midshaft of the femur. The incision is made along the line of fusion of the fascia lata and the cranial edge of the biceps femoris muscle.

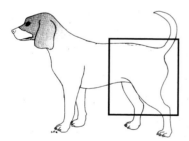

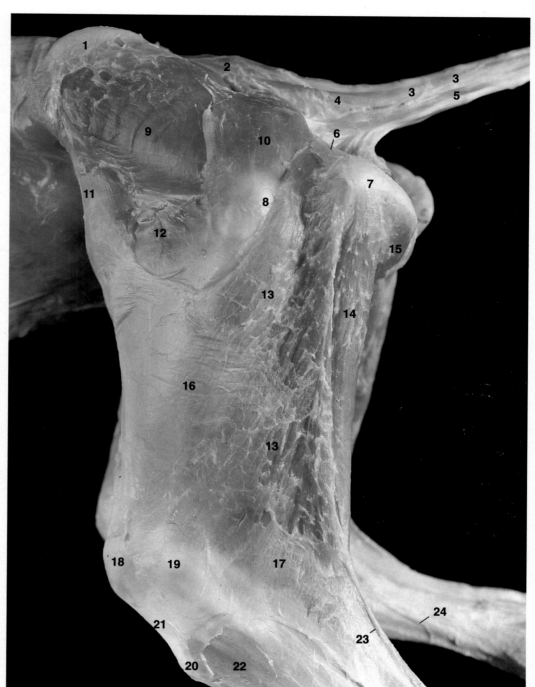

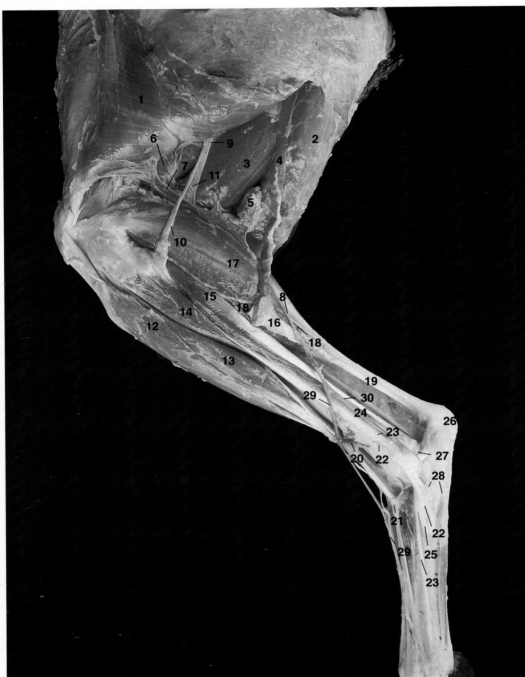

293 Lateral aspect of the left thigh, crus and tarsal region of a dog. The biceps femoris muscle has been reflected to reveal the division of the ischiatic nerve.

1	M. biceps femoris (reflected)
2	M. semitendinosus
3	M. semimembranosus
4	M. abductor cruris caudalis
5	Popliteal lymph node
6	Femoral artery and vein
7	Caudal femoral artery and vein
8	Lateral saphenous vein
9	Ischiatic nerve
10	Common peroneal (fibular) nerve
11	Tibial nerve
12	M. tibialis cranialis
13	M. extensor digitorum longus
14	M. peroneus longus
15	M. flexor hallucis longus (lateral head of M. flexor digitorum profundus)
16	Tendons of 1 and 2
17	M. gastrocnemius
18	M. flexor digitorum superficialis
19	Tendo calcaneus communis (Achilles)
20	Proximal extensor retinaculum
21	Distal extensor retinaculum
22	Tendon of 14
23	Tendon of M. extensor digitorum lateralis
24	M. peroneus brevis
25	Tendon of 24
26	Calcaneal tuberosity
27	Short part ⎱ of lateral collateral
28	Long part ⎰ ligament of tarsus
29	Cranial ramus ⎱ of lateral
30	Caudal ramus ⎰ saphenous vein

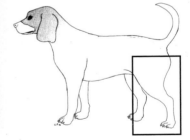

294 Lateral aspect of the pelvic and thigh regions of the left pelvic limb of a dog. The fascia lata and biceps femoris muscle have been removed to reveal the deeper muscles. The gluteal muscles have been reflected dorsally.

1	M. gluteus medius
2	M. gluteus superficialis } (cut)
3	M. gluteus profundus
4	M. piriformis
5	Hip joint capsule
6	M. sartorius
7	M. tensor fasciae latae
8	M. rectus femoris
9	M. vastus lateralis
10	Femur
11	M. quadratus femoris
12	Ischiatic nerve
13	Caudal gluteal artery and vein
14	M. adductor
15	M. semimembranosus
16	M. semitendinosus
17	M. abductor cruris caudalis (cut proximal end)
18	Common peroneal (fibular) nerve
19	Caudal cutaneous sural nerve
20	Tibial nerve
21	Lateral saphenous vein
22	Femoral artery and vein
23	Popliteal lymph node
24	M. gastrocnemius

• The tendons of insertion of the gluteal muscles onto or over the greater trochanter have been sectioned in the manner used in a dorsal surgical approach to the hip joint.

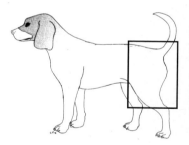

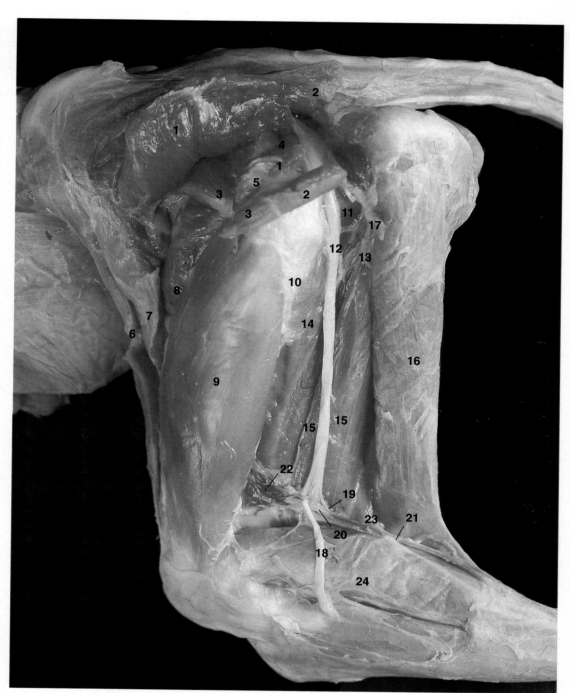

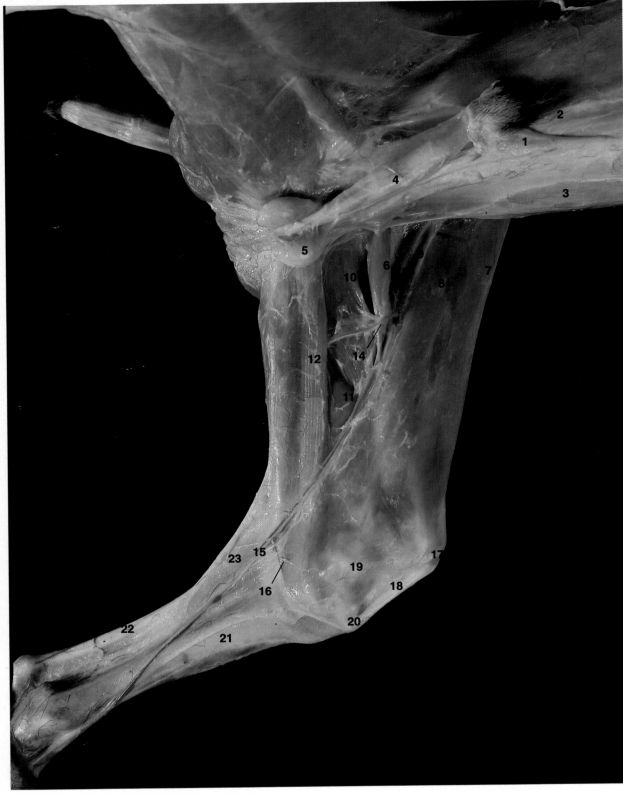

Medial aspect of the thigh region of the left pelvic limb of a dog, showing the superficial muscles.

1	M. preputialis
2	M. rectus abdominis
3	M. obliquus externus abdominis
4	Glans penis
5	Testes
6	M. pectineus
7	Cranial part ⎫ of M. sartorius
8	Caudal part ⎭
9	M. rectus femoris
10	Mm. adductores
11	M. semimembranosus
12	M. gracilis
13	Femoral triangle (with femoral artery, vein and saphenous nerve)
14	Muscular branches
15	Medial saphenous vein
16	Middle genicular vein
17	Patella
18	Patellar ligament
19	Medial epicondyle of femur
20	Tibial tuberosity
21	Body of tibia
22	Tendo calcaneus communis (Achilles)
23	M. gastrocnemius

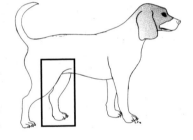

296 Medial aspect of the thigh region and crus of the left pelvic limb of a dog. The limb has been resected from its body attachments, and the caudal part of the sartorius muscle has been cut to reveal the deeper muscles.

1	M. sartorius
2	M. vastus medialis
3	M. adductor
4	M. semimembranosus
5	M. gracilis
6	M. semitendinosus
7	M. gastrocnemius
8	Saphenous artery, vein and nerve
9	M. popliteus
10	Medial collateral ligament of stifle
11	Patella
12	Patellar ligament
13	Tibial tuberosity
14	M. sartorius (cut end)
15	M. tibialis cranialis
16	M. flexor digitorum longus
17	M. flexor hallucis longus (lateral head of M. flexor digitorum profundus)
18	M. flexor digitorum superficialis
19	Tendons of 6 and M. biceps femoris (cut end)
20	Tendo calcaneus communis (Achilles)
21	Saphenous artery (caudal branch)
22	Tendon of 17
23	Tendon of 16
24	Body of tibia
25	Proximal extensor retinaculum
26	Tendon of 15
27	Medial collateral ligament of tarsus
28	Second metacarpal bone
29	Mm. interossei
30	Tendon of 18
31	Tendon of M. flexor digitorum profundus

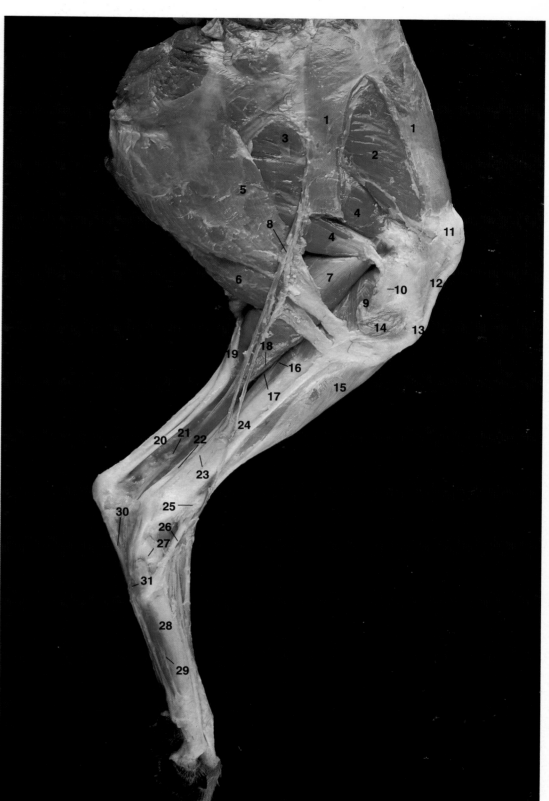

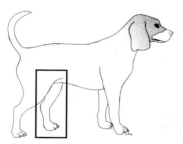

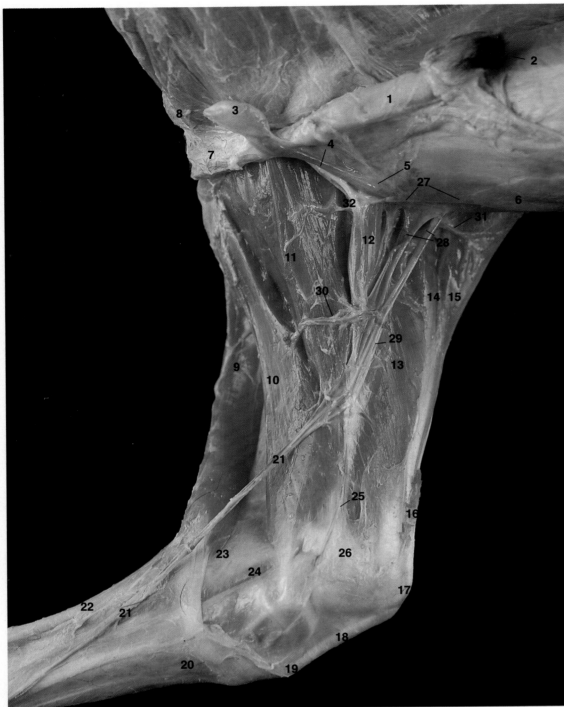

297 Medial aspect of the thigh region of the left pelvic limb of a dog. The gracilis and sartorius muscles have been resected.

1   Glans penis
2   External preputial orifice
3   Testis within parietal layer of vaginal tunic
4   Spermatic cord
5   Superficial (external) inguinal ring
6   M. obliquus externus abdominis
7   Body of penis
8   Ischiatic tuberosity
9   M. semitendinosus
10 M. semimembranosus
11 Mm. adductor magnus and brevis
12 M. pectineus
13 M. vastus medialis
14 M. rectus femoris
15 M. tensor fasciae latae
16 Fascia lata
17 Patella
18 Patellar ligament
19 Tibial tuberosity
20 Body of tibia
21 Medial saphenous artery and vein
22 Tendo calcaneus communis (Achilles)
23 M. gastrocnemius
24 M. popliteus
25 Middle genicular vein
26 Medial epicondyle of femur
27 Femoral triangle
28 Femoral artery and vein
29 Saphenous nerve (from femoral nerve)
30 Middle caudal femoral artery and vein
31 Branch of femoral nerve to 15 and M. sartorius
32 Branch of obturator nerve to M. pectineus and M. adductor

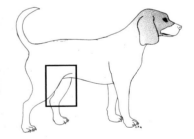

298 Medial aspect of the left crus of a dog.

1. M. semitendinosus
2. M. gastrocnemius
3. M. popliteus
4. Tendons of M. biceps femoris and 1 (cut end)
5. Saphenous artery and vein
6. M. flexor hallucis longus
7. M. flexor digitorum longus (medial head of M. flexor digitorum profundus)
8. Tendon of M. flexor hallucis longus (lateral head of M. flexor digitorum profundus)
9. M. tibialis cranialis
10. Body of tibia
11. Proximal extensor retinaculum
12. Tendo calcaneus communis (Achilles)
13. Calcaneal tuberosity
14. Tendon of M. tibialis caudalis
15. Medial collateral ligament
16. Tendon of M. flexor digitorum superficialis
17. Tendon of M. flexor digitorum profundus
18. Mm. interossei

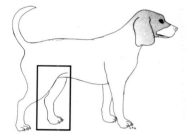

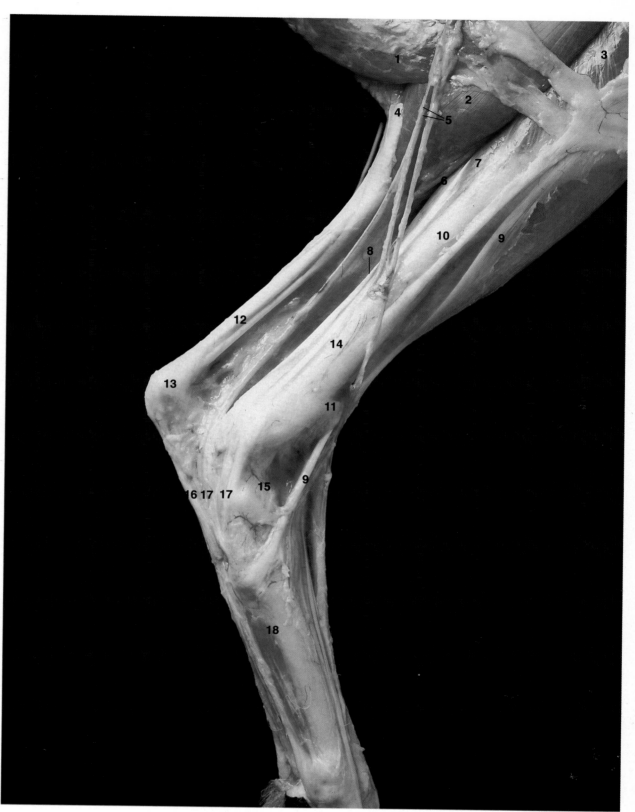

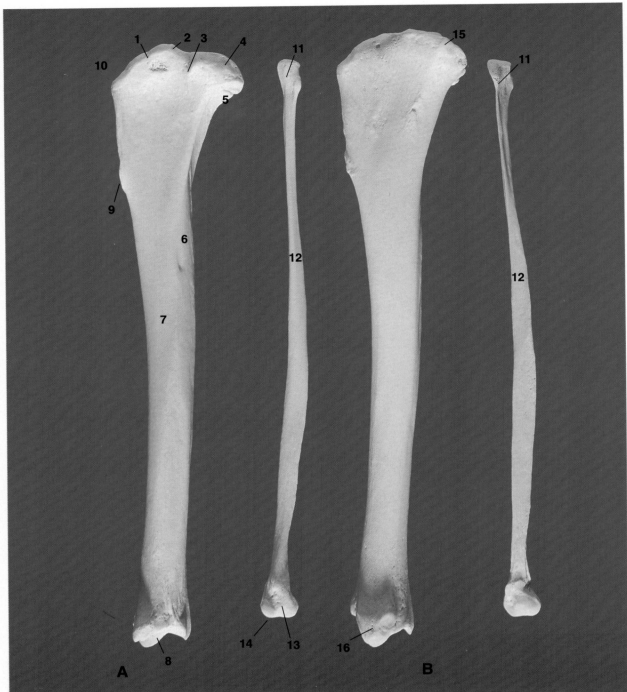

1	Cranial intercondylar area
2	Intercondylar eminence
3	Muscular (extensor) groove
4	Lateral condyle
5	Facet for articulation with fibula
6	Interosseous border
7	Body of tibia
8	Distal articular surface with cochlea of tibia
9	Cranial border (tibial crest)
10	Tibial tuberosity
11	Head } of fibula
12	Body
13	Lateral malleolus
14	Groove of 13
15	Medial condyle
16	Medial malleolus

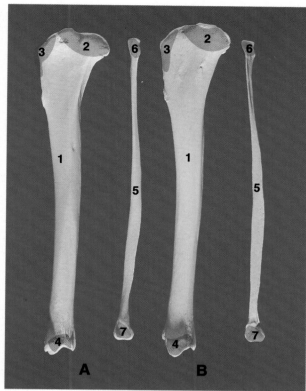

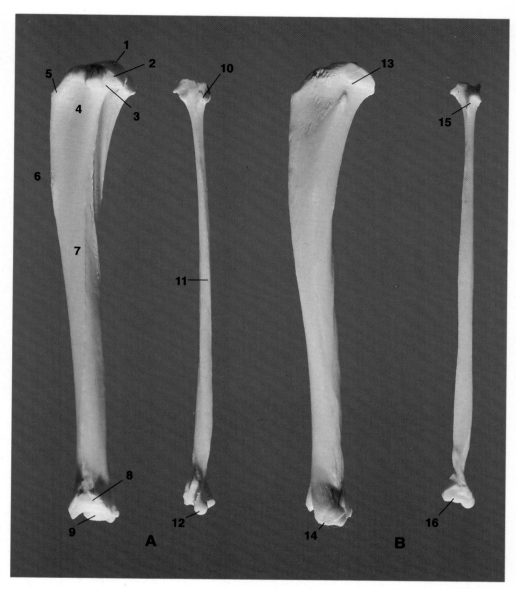

300 Lateral aspect of the left tibia and fibula (A) and medial aspect of the right tibia and fibula (B) of a dog, showing the centres of ossification.

1	Body of tibia
2	Proximal tibia
3	Tibial tuberosity
4	Distal tibia
5	Body of fibula
6	Proximal fibula
7	Distal fibula

301 Lateral aspect of the left tibia and fibula (A) and medial aspect of the right tibia and fibula (B) of a cat.

1	Intercondylar eminence	9	Distal articular surface
2	Lateral condyle of tibia	10	Head } of fibula
3	Facet for proximal articulation with fibula	11	Body
4	Muscular groove	12	Lateral malleolus
5	Tibial tuberosity	13	Medial condyle of tibia
6	Cranial border (tibial crest)	14	Medial malleolus
7	Body of tibia	15	Facet for proximal articulation with tibia
8	Facet for distal articulation with fibula	16	Facet for distal articulation with tibia

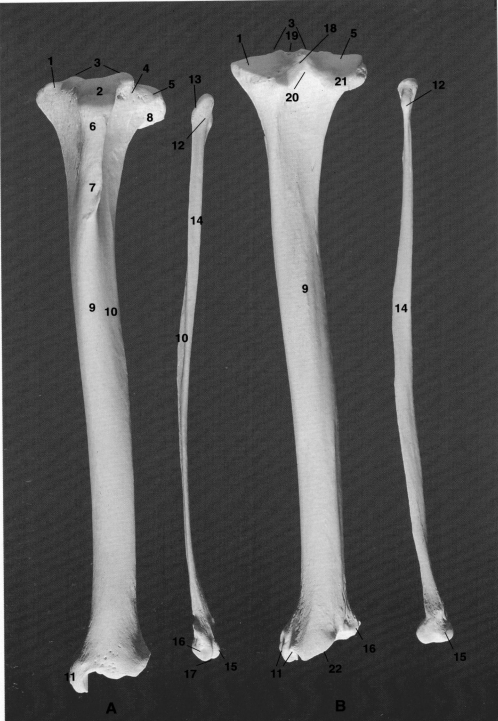

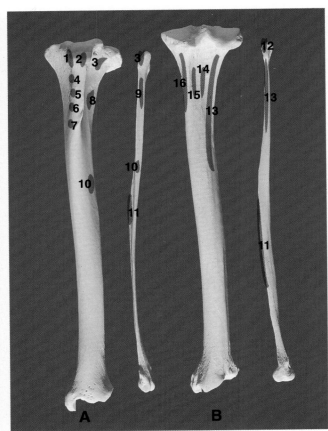

303 Cranial aspect of the left tibia and fibula (A) and caudal aspect of the right tibia and fibula (B) of a dog, showing areas of muscle attachment.

1	Biceps femoris
2	Cranial tibial
3	Peroneus longus
4	Quadriceps femoris
5	Sartorius
6	Gracilis
7	Semitendinosus
8	Flexor hallucis longus (radial)
9	Extensor digitorum lateralis
10	Extensor hallucis longus (ulnar)
11	Peroneus brevis
12	Caudal tibial (ulnar)
13	Flexor hallucis longus (lateral head of M. flexor digitorum profundus)
14	Caudal tibial (tibial)
15	Flexor digitorum longus (medial head of M. flexor digitorum profundus)
16	Popliteus

302 Cranial aspect of the left tibia and fibula (A) and caudal aspect of the right tibia and fibula (B) of a dog.

1	Medial condyle	9	Body of tibia	17	Groove of lateral malleolus (sulcus malleolaris lateralis)
2	Cranial intercondylar area	10	Interosseous border	18	Intercondylar eminence
3	Medial and lateral intercondylar tubercles	11	Medial malleolus	19	Caudal intercondylar area
4	Muscular (extensor) groove	12	Head of fibula	20	Popliteal notch
5	Lateral condyle	13	Facet for proximal articulation with fibula	21	Facet for articulation of sesamoid in tendon M. popliteus
6	Tibial tuberosity	14	Body of fibula	22	Distal articular surface with cochlea of tibia
7	Cranial border (tibial crest)	15	Lateral malleolus		
8	Facies articularis fibularis	16	Facies articulares malleoli		

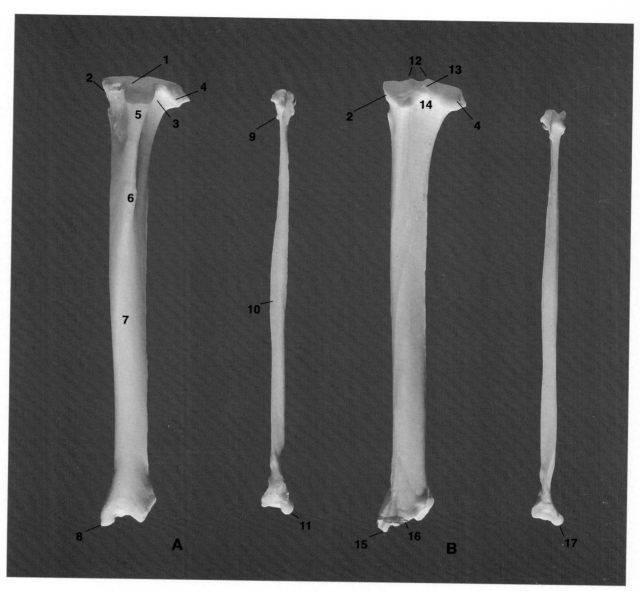

304 Cranial aspect of the left tibia and fibula (A) and caudal aspect of the right tibia and fibula (B) of a cat.

1	Cranial intercondylar area	7	Body of tibia	13	Caudal intercondylar area
2	Medial condyle	8	Medial malleolus	14	Popliteal notch
3	Muscular groove	9	Head } of fibula	15	Medial malleolus of tibia
4	Lateral condyle	10	Body	16	Distal articular surface
5	Tibial tuberosity	11	Lateral malleolus	17	Lateral malleolus of fibula
6	Cranial border	12	Intercondylar eminence		

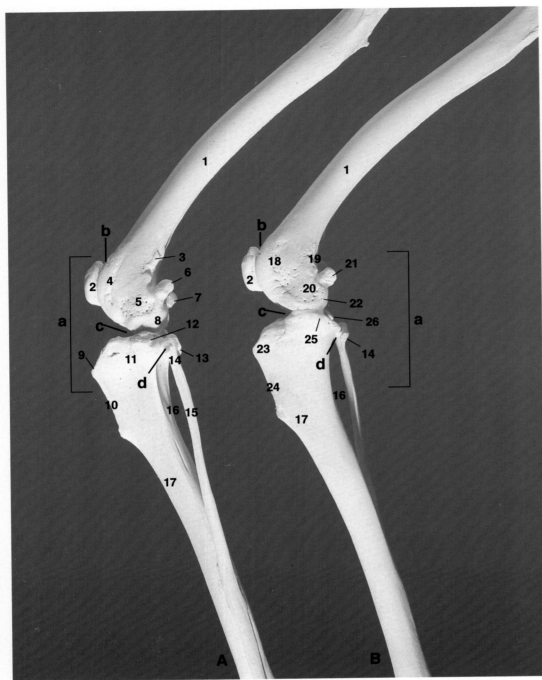

Lateral aspect of the left stifle joint and medial aspect of the right stifle joint of a dog.

a   Stifle joint
b   Femoropatellar joint
c   Femorotibial joint
d   Proximal tibiofibular joint

1   Body of femur
2   Patella
3   Lateral supracondylar tuberosity
4   Lateral ridge of trochlea
5   Lateral epicondyle
6   Lateral fabella ⎱ (in origin of M.
7   Medial fabella ⎰ gastrocnemius)
8   Lateral condyle of femur
9   Tibial tuberosity
10 Cranial border (tibial crest)
11 Muscular (extensor) groove
12 Lateral condyle of tibia
13 Proximal tibiofibular joint
14 Head ⎱ of fibula
15 Body ⎰
16 Interosseous space
17 Body of tibia
18 Medial ridge of trochlea
19 Medial supracondylar tuberosity
20 Medial epicondyle
21 Medial fabella (M. gastrocnemius)
22 Medial condyle of femur
23 Tibial crest
24 Cranial border
25 Medial condyle of tibia
26 Sesamoid tendon of M. popliteus

306 Cranial aspect of the left stifle joint (A) and caudal aspect of the right stifle joint (B) of a dog.

a	Stifle joint
b	Femoropatellar joint
c	Femorotibial joint
d	Proximal tibiofibular joint

1	Body of femur
2	Patella
3	Medial ridge } of trochlea
4	Lateral ridge } of trochlea
5	Medial epicondyle } of femur
6	Lateral epicondyle } of femur
7	Medial condyle } of femur
8	Lateral condyle } of femur
9	Medial condyle } of tibia
10	Lateral condyle } of tibia
11	Intercondylar area
12	Tibial tuberosity
13	Cranial border (tibial crest)
14	Head } of fibula
15	Body } of fibula
16	Interosseous space
17	Body of tibia
18	Medial and lateral supracondylar tuberosities
19	Medial and lateral fabellae (in origin of M. gastrocnemius)
20	Popliteal surface
21	Sesamoid in tendon of M. popliteus
22	Intercondylar fossa of femur
23	Caudal intercondylar area
24	Proximal tibiofibular joint

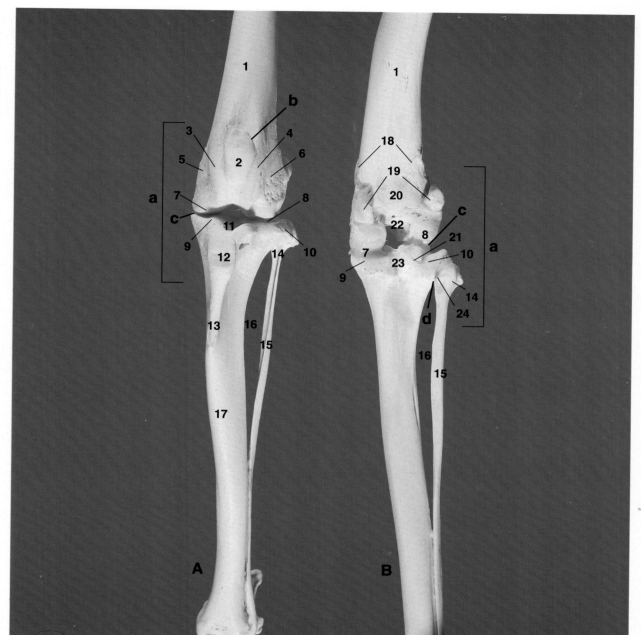

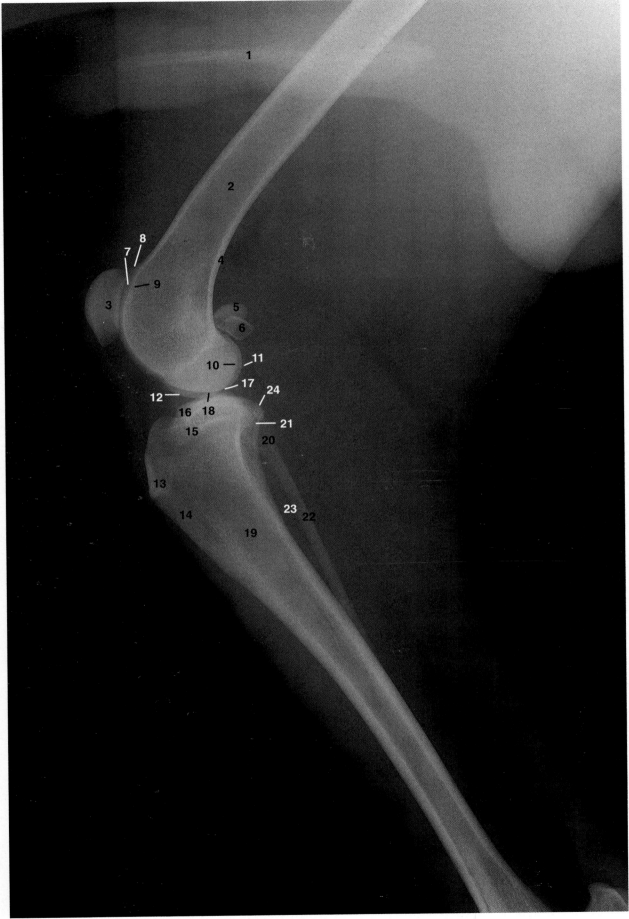

1	Os penis
2	Body of femur
3	Patella
4	Lateral supracondylar tuberosity
5	Lateral fabella ⎫ (in origin of M.
6	Medial fabella ⎭ gastrocnemius)
7	femoropatellar joint
8	lateral ridge ⎫ of trochlea
9	Medial ridge ⎭
10	Lateral condyle ⎫ of femur
11	Medial condyle ⎭
12	Femorotibial joint
13	Tibial tuberosity
14	Cranial border (tibial crest)
15	Lateral condyle ⎫ of tibia
16	Medial condyle ⎭
17	Lateral intercondylar tubercle
18	Medial intercondylar tubercle
19	Body of tibia
20	Head of fibula
21	Proximal tibiofibular joint
22	Body of fibula
23	Interosseous space
24	Fabella in the tendon of M. popliteus

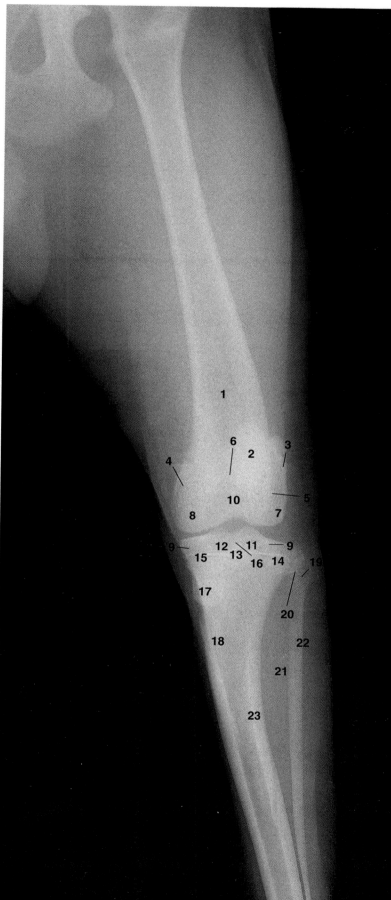

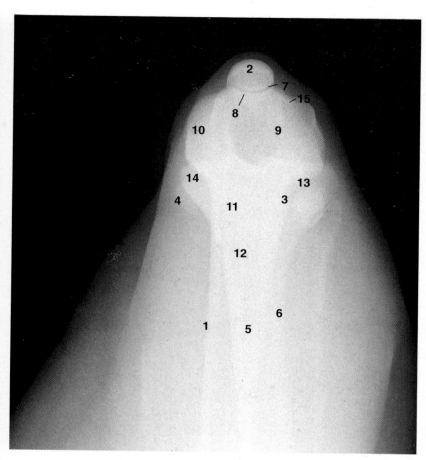

308 Craniocaudal radiograph of the stifle joint of a dog.

309 Radiograph of the flexed stifle joint of a dog.

1	Body of femur
2	Patella
3	Lateral fabella ⎫ (in origin of M.
4	Medial fabella ⎭ gastrocnemius)
5	Lateral ridge ⎫ of trochlea
6	Medial ridge ⎭
7	Lateral condyle ⎫ of femur
8	Medial condyle ⎭
9	Femorotibial joint space
10	Intercondylar fossa
11	Lateral intercondylar tubercle
12	Medial intercondylar tubercle
13	Intercondylar area
14	Lateral condyle ⎫ of tibia
15	Medial condyle ⎭
16	Fabella in tendon of M. popliteus
17	Tibial tuberosity
18	Base of tibial crest
19	Head of fibula
20	Proximal tibiofibular joint
21	Interosseous space
22	Body of fibula
23	Body of tibia

1	Body of femur
2	Patella
3	Lateral fabella ⎫ (in origin of M.
4	Medial fabella ⎭ gastrocnemius)
5	Body of tibia
6	Body of fibula
7	Femoropatellar joint
8	Trochlear groove
9	Lateral condyle ⎫ of femur
10	Medial condyle ⎭
11	Tibial tuberosity
12	Cranial border (tibial crest)
13	Lateral condyle ⎫ of tibia
14	Medial condyle ⎭
15	Extensor fossa

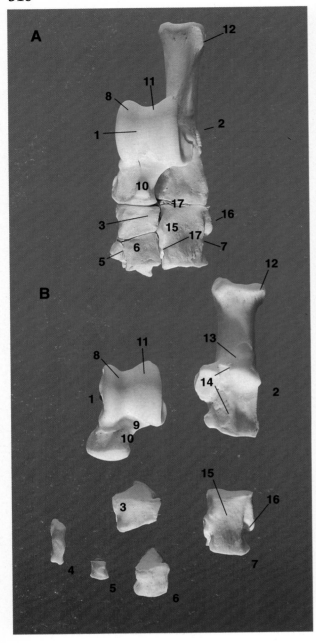

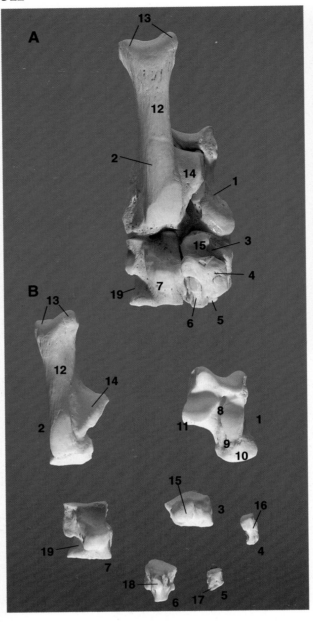

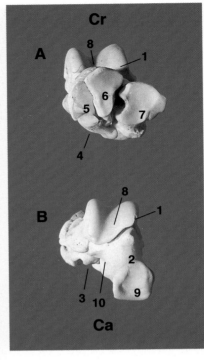

312 Distal aspect of the left tarsus (A) and proximal aspect of the right tarsus (B) of a dog. Cranial (Cr) and caudal (Ca) orientations are indicated.

1	Talus
2	Calcaneus
3	Central
4	First
5	Second } tarsal bone
6	Third
7	Fourth
8	Proximal trochlea
9	Calcaneal tuberosity
10	Sustentaculum tali

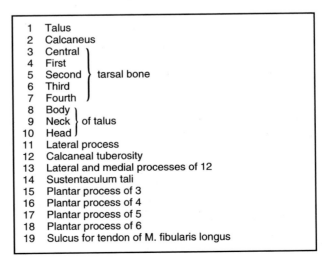

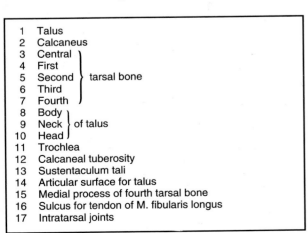

311 Plantar aspect of the articulated (A) and separated (B) left tarsus of a dog.

310 Dorsal aspect of the articulated (A) and separated (B) left tarsus of a dog.

1	Talus
2	Calcaneus
3	Central
4	First
5	Second } tarsal bone
6	Third
7	Fourth
8	Body
9	Neck } of talus
10	Head
11	Trochlea
12	Calcaneal tuberosity
13	Sustentaculum tali
14	Articular surface for talus
15	Medial process of fourth tarsal bone
16	Sulcus for tendon of M. fibularis longus
17	Intratarsal joints

1	Talus
2	Calcaneus
3	Central
4	First
5	Second } tarsal bone
6	Third
7	Fourth
8	Body
9	Neck } of talus
10	Head
11	Lateral process
12	Calcaneal tuberosity
13	Lateral and medial processes of 12
14	Sustentaculum tali
15	Plantar process of 3
16	Plantar process of 4
17	Plantar process of 5
18	Plantar process of 6
19	Sulcus for tendon of M. fibularis longus

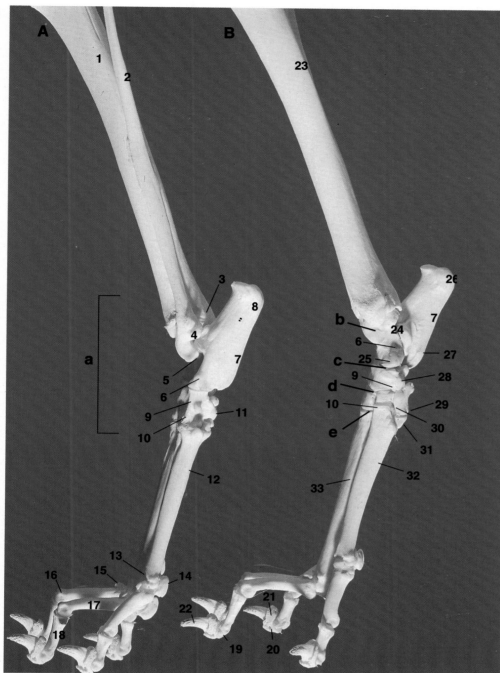

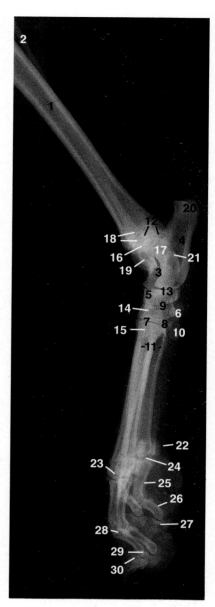

314 Mediolateral radiograph of the tarsal joint and pes of a dog.

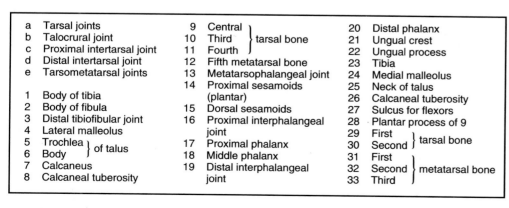

313 Lateral aspect of the left tarsus and pes (A) and medial aspect of the right tarsus and pes (B) of a dog.

a	Tarsal joints	9	Central ⎫	20	Distal phalanx
b	Talocrural joint	10	Third ⎬ tarsal bone	21	Ungual crest
c	Proximal intertarsal joint	11	Fourth ⎭	22	Ungual process
d	Distal intertarsal joint	12	Fifth metatarsal bone	23	Tibia
e	Tarsometatarsal joints	13	Metatarsophalangeal joint	24	Medial malleolus
		14	Proximal sesamoids (plantar)	25	Neck of talus
1	Body of tibia			26	Calcaneal tuberosity
2	Body of fibula	15	Dorsal sesamoids	27	Sulcus for flexors
3	Distal tibiofibular joint	16	Proximal interphalangeal joint	28	Plantar process of 9
4	Lateral malleolus	17	Proximal phalanx	29	First ⎫ tarsal bone
5	Trochlea ⎫ of talus	18	Middle phalanx	30	Second ⎭
6	Body ⎭	19	Distal interphalangeal joint	31	First ⎫
7	Calcaneus			32	Second ⎬ metatarsal bone
8	Calcaneal tuberosity			33	Third ⎭

1	Body of tibia	17	Medial malleolus
2	Body of fibula	18	Cochlea of tibia
3	Talus	19	Trochlea of talus
4	Calcaneus	20	Calcaneal tuberosity
5	Central ⎫	21	Sustenaculum tali
6	First ⎬	22	Proximal sesamoids
7	Second ⎬ tarsal bone	23	Dorsal sesamoid
8	Third ⎬	24	Metatarsophalangeal joint
9	Fourth ⎭		
10	First metatarsal bone	25	Proximal phalanx
11	Second to fifth metatarsal bones	26	Middle phalanx
		27	Distal phalanx
12	Talocrural joint	28	Proximal interphalangeal joint
13	Proximal intertarsal joint		
14	Distal intertarsal joint	29	Distal interphalangeal joint
15	Tarsometatarsal joint		
16	Lateral malleolus	30	Ungual crest

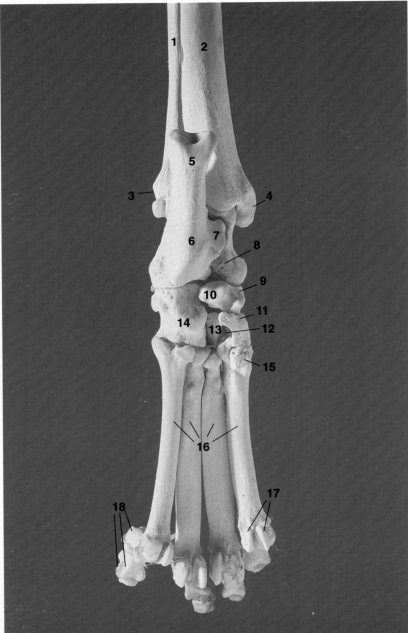

315 Plantar aspect of the tarsal joint and pes of a dog.

1	Fibula	11	First
2	Tibia	12	Second
3	Lateral malleolus	13	Third
4	Medial malleolus	14	Fourth
5	Calcaneal tuberosity	15	First metatarsal bone
6	Calcaneus	16	Second to fifth metatarsal bones
7	Sustentaculum tali	17	Proximal sesamoids
8	Talus	18	Proximal, middle and distal
9	Central tarsal bone		phalanges
10	Plantar process of 9		

(12, 13, 14 grouped as: tarsal bone)

316 Dorsoplantar radiograph of the tarsal joint and pes of a dog.

1	Body of tibia
2	Body of fibula
3	Talus
4	Calcaneus
5	Central
6	First
7	Second } tarsal bone
8	Third
9	Fourth
10	First
11	Second
12	Third } metatarsal bone
13	Fourth
14	Fifth
15	Talocrural joint
16	Proximal intertarsal joint
17	Distal intertarsal joint
18	Tarsometatarsal joint
19	Lateral malleolus
20	Medial malleolus
21	Dorsal border
22	Lateral groove } of cochlea
23	Medial groove } of tibia
24	Lateral ridge } of trochlea
25	Medial ridge } of talus
26	Groove
27	Calcaneal tuberosity
28	Sustentaculum tali
29	Proximal sesamoids
30	Metatarsophalangeal joint
31	Outline of metatarsal pad
32	Proximal phalanx
33	Proximal interphalangeal joint
34	Middle phalanx
35	Distal interphalangeal joint
36	Distal phalanx
37	Ungual crest
38	Ungual process

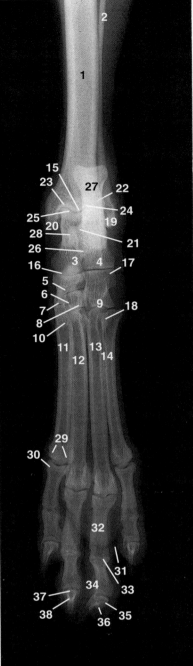

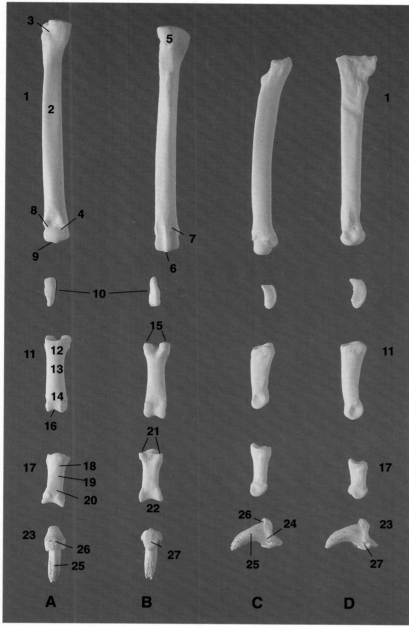

318 Dorsal aspect of a typical digit in the pes of a dog, showing the centres of ossification.

1	Body of metatarsal bone
2	Distal
3	Body of proximal phalanx
4	Proximal
5	Body of middle phalanx
6	Proximal
7	Body of distal phalanx

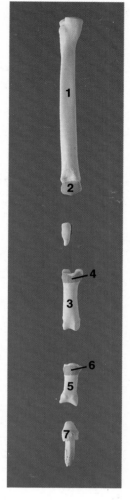

317 Dorsal (A), plantar (B), abaxial (C) and axial (D) aspects of a typical digit in the pes of a dog.

1	Metatarsal bone		17	Middle phalanx
2	Body		18	Base
3	Base	of 1	19	Body
4	Head		20	Head of 17
5	Plantar tubercles		21	Plantar tubercles
6	Sagittal crest		22	Trochlea
7	Proximal sesamoid impression		23	Distal phalanx
8	Dorsal sesamoid fossa		24	Body of 23
9	Trochlea of 1		25	Ungual process
10	Proximal sesamoid		26	Ungual crest
11	Proximal phalanx		27	Insertion of M. flexor digitorum profundus
12	Base			
13	Body			
14	Head	of 11		
15	Plantar tubercles			
16	Trochlea			

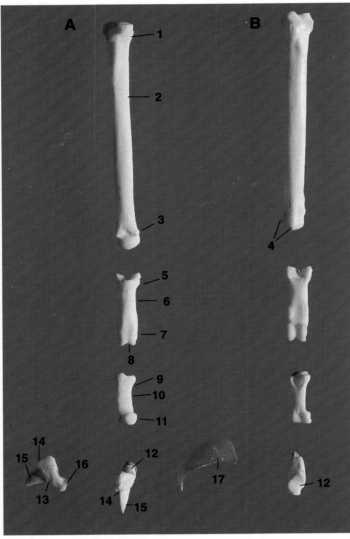

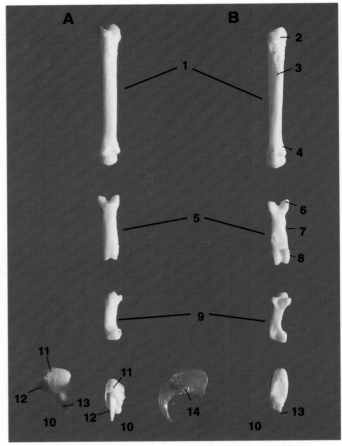

319 Dorsal (A) and plantar (B) aspects of a typical digit in the pes of a cat. The lateral aspects of the distal phalanx and the claw are also displayed.

1	Base ⎫		12	Base ⎫ of distal phalanx
2	Body ⎬ of metatarsal bone		13	Body ⎭
3	Head ⎭		14	Ungual crest
4	Sesamoid impression		15	Ungual process
5	Base ⎫		16	Tubercle for insertion of M.
6	Body ⎬ of proximal phalanx			flexor digitorum profundus
7	Head ⎭		17	Claw (unguis)
8	Trochlea			
9	Base ⎫			
10	Body ⎬ of middle phalanx			
11	Head ⎭			

320 Dorsal (A) and palmar (B) aspects of a typical digit in the manus of a cat. The lateral aspects of the distal phalanx and the claw are also displayed.

1	Metacarpal bone
2	Base ⎫
3	Body ⎬ of metacarpal bone
4	Head ⎭
5	Proximal phalanx
6	Base ⎫
7	Body ⎬ of first phalanx
8	Head ⎭
9	Middle phalanx
10	Distal phalanx
11	Ungual crest
12	Ungual process
13	Tubercle for insertion of M. flexor digitorum profundus
14	Claw (unguis)

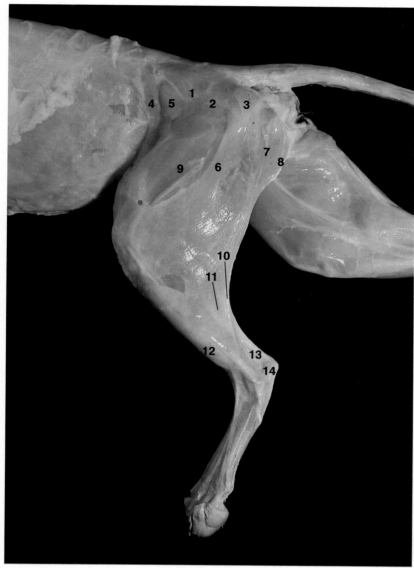

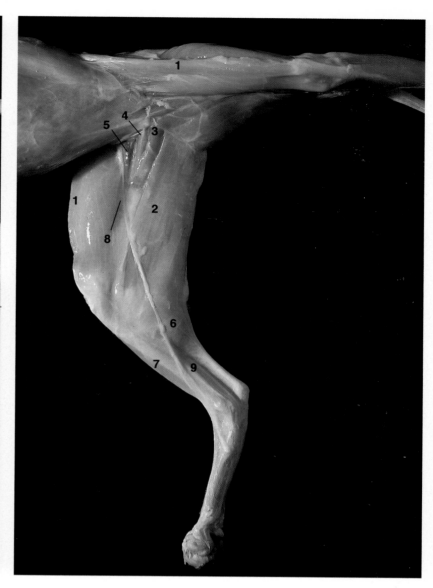

321 Lateral aspect of the pelvic limb of a cat, showing the superficial muscles.

1	M. gluteus medius	9	M. quadriceps (vastus lateralis)
2	M. gluteus superficialis	10	Saphenous vein
3	M. caudofemoralis	11	M. soleus
4	M. sartorius	12	M. tibialis cranialis
5	M. tensor fasciae latae	13	Tendo calcaneus communis
6	M. biceps femoris		(Achilles)
7	M. semitendinosus	14	Calcaneal tuberosity
8	M. semimembranosus		

322 Medial aspect of the pelvic limb of a cat, showing the superficial muscles.

1	M. sartorius		artery, vein and saphenous nerve)
2	M. gracilis	6	M. gastrocnemius
3	M. adductor	7	M. tibialis cranialis
4	M. pectineus	8	Saphenous vein
5	Femoral triangle (with femoral	9	M. flexor digitorum profundus

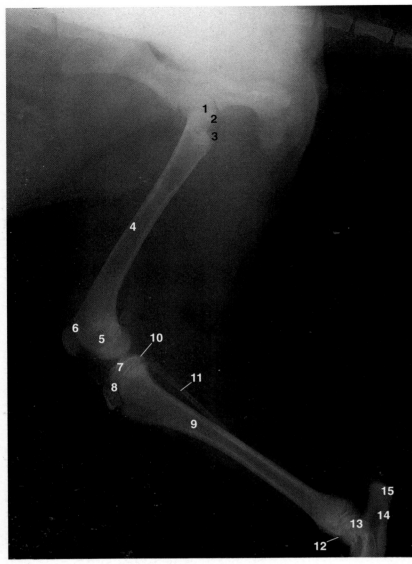

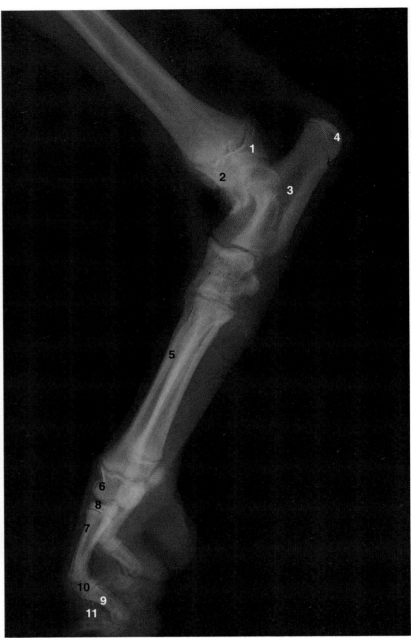

323 Mediolateral radiograph of the thigh region, stifle and tarsal joint of a puppy, showing the centres of ossification.

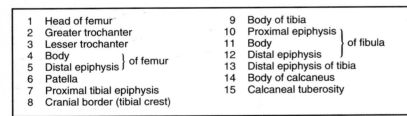

1	Head of femur	9	Body of tibia
2	Greater trochanter	10	Proximal epiphysis ⎫
3	Lesser trochanter	11	Body ⎬ of fibula
4	Body ⎫ of femur	12	Distal epiphysis ⎭
5	Distal epiphysis ⎬	13	Distal epiphysis of tibia
6	Patella	14	Body of calcaneus
7	Proximal tibial epiphysis	15	Calcaneal tuberosity
8	Cranial border (tibial crest)		

324 Mediolateral radiograph of the tarsal joint and pes of a puppy, showing the centres of ossification.

1	Distal epiphysis of tibia	7	Body ⎫ of proximal
2	Distal epiphysis of fibula	8	Proximal epiphysis ⎬ phalanx
3	Body of calcaneus	9	Body ⎫ of middle
4	Calcaneal tuberosity	10	Proximal epiphysis ⎬ phalanx
5	Body ⎫ of metatarsus	11	Body of distal phalanx
6	Distal epiphysis ⎬		

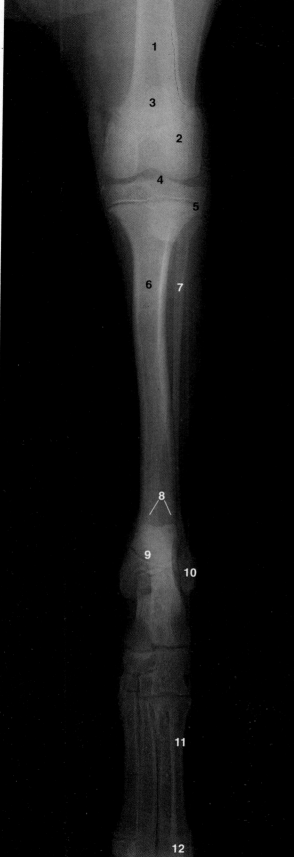

325 Craniocaudal dorsoplantar radiograph of the stifle and tarsal joint of a puppy, showing the centres of ossification.

1	Body	} of femur
2	Distal epiphysis	
3	Patella	
4	Proximal epiphysis of tibia	
5	Proximal epiphysis of fibula	
6	Body of tibia	
7	Body of fibula	
8	Calcaneal tuberosity	
9	Distal epiphysis of tibia	
10	Distal epiphysis of fibula	
11	Body	} of metatarsus
12	Distal epiphysis	

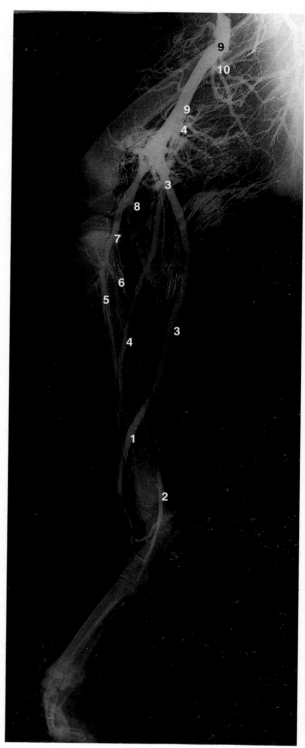

326 Mediolateral radiograph of a venogram of the pelvic limb of a dog.

1	Cranial branch	⎞ of lateral
2	Caudal branch	⎠ saphenous vein
3	Lateral saphenous vein	
4	Medial saphenous vein	
5	Cranial tibial vein	
6	Caudal tibial vein	
7	Popliteal vein	
8	Distal caudal femoral vein	
9	Femoral vein	
10	Deep femoral vein	

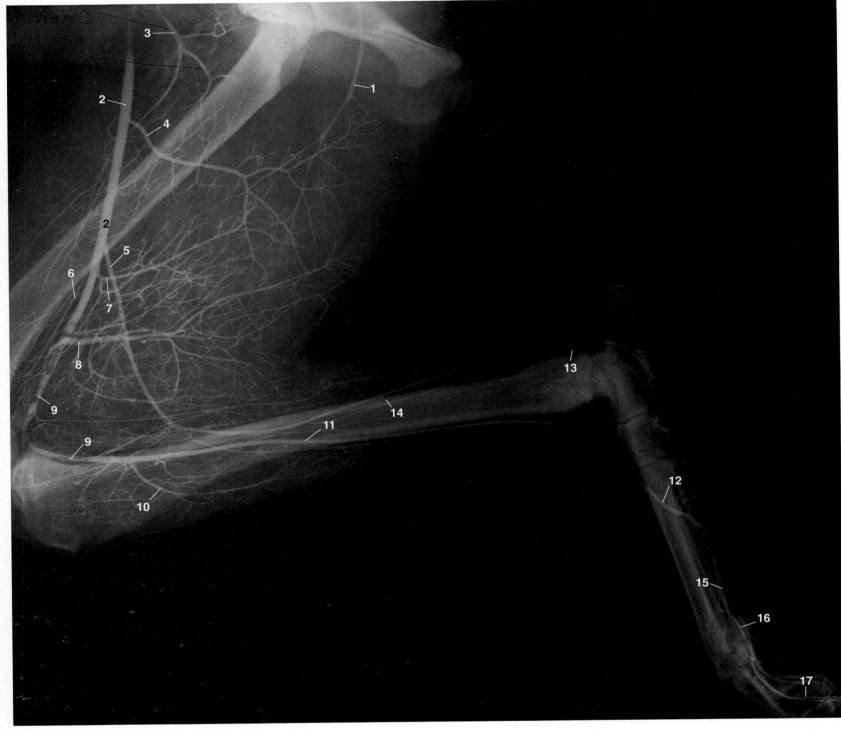

327 Mediolateral radiograph of an arteriogram of the pelvic limb of a dog.

1	Caudal gluteal artery from internal iliac artery	9	Popliteal artery
2	Femoral artery from external iliac artery	10	Caudal tibial artery
3	Lateral circumflex femoral artery	11	Cranial tibial artery
4	Proximal caudal femoral artery	12	Perforating metatarsal artery
5	Saphenous artery	13	Caudal branch ⎫ of 5
6	Descending genicular artery	14	Cranial branch ⎭
7	Middle caudal femoral artery	15	Plantar metatarsal arteries
8	Distal caudal femoral artery	16	Plantar common digital arteries
		17	Plantar proper digitial arteries

Index

Numbers refer to figures.
References are to adult dogs, unless otherwise stated.